MILADY'S STANDARD
FUNDAMENTALS
FOR ESTHETICIANS
WORKBOOK

To be used with
MILADY'S STANDARD FUNDAMENTALS FOR ESTHETICIANS

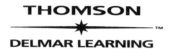

Milady's Standard Fundamentals for Estheticians Workbook

For permission to use material from this text or product, contact us by
Tel   (800) 730-2214
Fax   (800) 730-2215
www.thomsonrights.com

Library of Congress Catalog Card Number: 2002074216
ISBN 1-56253-837-3

NOTICE TO THE READER

MILADY'S STANDARD
FUNDAMENTALS
FOR ESTHETICIANS
WORKBOOK

To be used with
MILADY'S STANDARD FUNDAMENTALS FOR ESTHETICIANS

THOMSON

™

DELMAR LEARNING   AUSTRALIA   CANADA   MEXICO   SINGAPORE   SPAIN   UNITED KINGDOM   UNITED STATES

CONTENTS

How to Use This Workbook

This workbook has been especially designed to meet the needs, interests, and abilities of students receiving training for a career in esthetics, the art of skin care. It has been organized to be used in conjunction with *Milady's Standard Fundamentals for Estheticians, 9E.*

The material presented here has been prepared in accordance with the accepted methods of vocational training that are approved by state licensing organizations. All materials have been compiled with the assistance of leading educators and teachers in the field of esthetics and cosmetology.

1. **Assignment of the Lesson**

   Pages to be read and studied are listed at the top of the page.

2. **Learning the Lesson**

   The student writes the answers in the workbook, consulting the text and glossary/index located in the back of *Milady's Standard Fundamentals for Estheticians, 9E.*

3. **Correction of the Lesson**

   Answers may be corrected and rated during class discussions.

4. **Review of the Lesson**

   Various tests emphasize the essential facts and measure the student's progress.

1

SKIN CARE HISTORY AND OPPORTUNITIES

Date: _____

Rating: _____

Text pages: 2–17

TOPIC 1: THE HISTORY OF GROOMING AND SKIN CARE

1. In ancient times, people around the world used pigments on their hair, skin, and nails made from materials such as _____ .

2. Who were the first people to use distillation to extract essential oils? _____

3. From what language do the words *cosmetics* and *cosmetology* come? _____

4. Cold cream was made more stable in the early twentieth century when natural vegetable oil was replaced with _____ .

5. The _____ are most famous for their public baths.

6. The period in European history between classical antiquity and the Renaissance is called _____ _____ .

7. One of the most austere periods in history, during which the use of makeup was discouraged, spanned the reign of _____ .

8. Women during the 1920s were influenced in their hairstyles and makeup by _____ .

9. In the 1970s and 1980s, there was a new surge of interest in _____ .

10. During the last two decades of the twentieth century, _____ sprang up all over the country, featuring services that integrated beauty and wellness.

RAPID REVIEW TEST

Date: _____

Rating: _____

Insert the correct term in the space provided.

aromatics	henna	nutriceuticals
cold cream	kohl	techniceuticals
cosmeceuticals	*kosmetikos*	vermilion
full-service salon		

1. Ancient Egyptians used _____ , a metallic substance related to arsenic and tin, as eye makeup.

2. _____ is a dye derived from the mignonette tree and used to tint the hair.

3. Frankincense, myrrh, cinnamon, and rosemary, which are _____ , were used by the Hebrews in anointing and healing the sick.

4. The words *cosmetics* and *cosmetology* are derived from the word _____.

5. The first modern cosmetic compound is considered to be _____.

6. The brilliant red pigment used by Greek women to color their cheeks and lips is called _____.

7. A _____ offers hair care, hairstyling, and a full range of grooming and beauty services.

8. Cosmetics with therapeutic properties are called _____.

9. Internal supplements that aid the health of the skin from the inside are _____.

10. Anti-aging procedures such as microdermabrasion are called _____.

TOPIC 2: CAREER OPPORTUNITIES

1. What is the meaning of the word *esthetics?* _____

_____

2. Estheticians offer skin care treatments and sell cosmetics but cannot _____

or _____.

3. Name five responsibilities of an esthetician in a cosmetic surgeon's office:

   a) _____

   b) _____

   c) _____

   d) _____

   e) _____

4. Name five responsibilities of an esthetician in a dermatologist's office:

   a) _____

   b) _____

   c) _____

   d) _____

   e) _____

5. Spider vein removal, hair reduction, and wrinkle treatments are performed in a _____.

6. Manufacturers of cosmetics often hire _____
   to call on salons or stores to sell products and build clientele.

7. Cosmetics _____ work for department stores, salons, or specialty businesses and travel
   frequently to trade shows and manufacturers' showrooms.

8. Educators may teach esthetics in _____ , _____ ,
   _____ , or _____ high schools.

9. The decade in which modern esthetics came of age is considered to be the _____.

10. Skin care in general is becoming more _____ than corrective.

RAPID REVIEW TEST

Date: _____

Rating: _____

Insert the correct term in the space provided.

baby boomers   medical esthetics

camouflage therapy   medi-spa

education directors   restorative art

esthetics   state board members

1. The branch of anatomical science dealing with the health and well-being of the skin is _____.

2. The field that integrates surgical and esthetic treatments is called _____.

3. The medical setting in which patients receive both spa services and surgical procedures is called a _____.

4. When you apply makeup to cover scars or congenital defects, you are performing _____.

5. A makeup artist who works in a mortuary is skilled at _____.

6. Manufacturers often employ estheticians as _____, who conduct seminars and workshops, display products at conventions, and talk with teachers.

7. Licensing exams are conducted and licenses are granted by _____.

8. Americans born between 1946 and 1964 are known as _____.

2

YOUR PROFESSIONAL IMAGE

Date: _____

Rating: _____

Text pages: 18–34

TOPIC 1: YOUR PROFESSIONAL APPEARANCE

1. The impression you project as a person engaged in the profession of esthetics is your _____ _____ .

2. Your professional image is made up of your _____ and your _____ in the workplace.

3. You can achieve balance and health by:

   a) _____

   b) _____

   c) _____

   d) _____

4. Personal hygiene is the daily maintenance of _____ and _____ through certain sanitary practices.

5. Personal hygiene consists of certain basic tasks, including:

   a) _____

   b) _____

   c) _____

   d) _____

   e) _____

   f) _____

6. Unused makeup should be discarded every _____ .

7. Your posture, movements, and the way you walk make up your _____ .

8. Good posture can prevent _____ and other physical problems.

9. To achieve good standing posture, practice these seven steps:

   a) _____

   b) _____

   c) _____

   d) _____

   e) _____

   f) _____

   g) _____

10. To achieve good sitting posture, take these four steps:

   a) _____

   b) _____

   c) _____

   d) _____

TOPIC 2: PROFESSIONAL CONDUCT

1. You may not be able to change an inborn characteristic or a genetic trait, but you can change your
   _____ .

2. Employers are interested in hiring people who have a strong _____
   —in other words, people who are committed to doing a good job.

3. To maintain a productive work environment, team players develop the right attitude, consisting of the following standards:

   a) _____   e) _____

   b) _____   f) _____

   c) _____   g) _____

   d) _____

4. If you consistently practice good _____
   techniques, you can decrease the potential for conflict with clients and coworkers.

5. An important rule when dealing with clients is never to engage in _____ .

RAPID REVIEW TEST

Date: _____

Rating: _____

Insert the correct term in the space provided.

attitude   discretion   sensitivity
diplomacy   emotional stability

1. When you do not share with others what your clients have told you in confidence, you are showing _____.

2. Your outlook, or _____, affects the way you live your life.

3. Showing concern and understanding for the feelings of others is a sign of _____.

4. Self-control is an important aspect of _____.

5. The skill of _____ involves being tactful in your dealings with other people.

TOPIC 3: PROFESSIONAL ETHICS

1. The moral principles by which we live and work are called _____.

2. The first step in establishing credibility as an esthetician is obtaining the appropriate _____.

3. General guidelines for becoming a confident, trustworthy professional are:

    a) _____

    b) _____

    c) _____

    d) _____

    e) _____

    f) _____

    g) _____
       _____

    h) _____

    i) _____

TOPIC 4: LIFE SKILLS

1. Some of the important life skills are:

   a) _____

   b) _____

   c) _____

   d) _____

   e) _____

   f) _____

   g) _____

   h) _____

   i) _____

   j) _____

   k) _____

   l) _____

   m) _____

2. Becoming a successful person depends in large part on building your _____, which is based on inner strength.

3. Three habits that can prevent you from being your most productive are:

   a) _____

   b) _____

   c) _____

4. Ownership of your own salon is an example of a _____ goal.

5. Making a list of tasks for the day, from most to least important, is a way of _____.

6. Good time management is essential to professional success. Which of the following contribute to the wise use of your time and energy?

_____ problem-solving techniques

_____ exercising once or twice a month

_____ to-do lists

_____ organizing your workday just before your first client

_____ scheduling as many appointments as possible

_____ asking new clients to arrive 10 minutes early

3

SANITATION AND DISINFECTION

Date: _____

Rating: _____

Text pages: 36–57

TOPIC 1: BACTERIA, VIRUSES, AND PARASITES

1. Why should estheticians study bacteria? _____

2. Tiny plant or animal cells that cannot be seen with the naked eye are called _____ .

3. Bacteria are also known as _____ or _____ .

4. _____ bacteria decompose garbage, improve soil fertility, and help digest food.

5. _____ bacteria cause disease in plant or animal tissue.

6. What are the shapes of the following bacteria?

    a) _____ cocci

    b) _____ bacilli

    c) _____ spirilla

7. Which bacteria cause the following diseases?

    a) _____ pustules and boils

    b) _____ tuberculosis

    c) _____ strep throat

    d) _____ Lyme disease

    e) _____ pneumonia

8. Identify the bacteria illustrated below:

    a) _____

    b) _____

    c) _____

a.

b.

c.

9. The life cycle of bacteria is made up of these two phases:

    a) _____

    b) _____

10. To survive difficult conditions such as famine or unsuitable temperatures, certain bacteria form _____ _____ .

11. What is one important difference between viruses and bacteria? _____ _____

12. Viruses are generally resistant to _____.

13. The HIV virus is transmitted through:

    a) _____

    b) _____

    c) _____

14. _____ is a viral disease characterized by liver inflammation.

15. In what ways does the body fight infection?

    a) _____

    b) _____

    c) _____

    d) _____

16. Pathogenic bacteria and viruses that are carried through the body in blood or body fluids are called

    _____.

17. When pathogenic bacteria or viruses invade the body, _____ may occur.

18. Pus is a fluid product of _____.

19. A disease that spreads by contact from one person to another is called _____.

20. A _____ infection is confined to a particular part of the body.

21. When bacteria or viruses are carried throughout the body, a _____ infection results.

22. _____ live in or on another living organism and draw their nourishment from that organism.

23. Ringworm and favus are caused by plant parasites or _____.

24. Head lice and itch mites are types of _____ parasites.

25. The ability of the body to resist infection is called _____.

RAPID REVIEW TEST

Date: _____

Rating: _____

Insert the correct term in the space provided.

acquired	HIV	nonpathogenic
contagious	host	pus
fungi	inoculation	scabies
general infection	microscope	spores
hepatitis	natural	viruses

1. The majority of bacteria are classified as _____.

2. The most resistant form of life on Earth is _____.

3. The common cold, smallpox, and AIDS are all caused by _____.

4. Bacteria become visible when observed under a _____.

5. _____ is the virus that causes AIDS.

6. A disease caused by a virus similar to HIV but more easily contracted than HIV is _____.

7. One sign of bacterial infection is _____.

8. Tuberculosis, ringworm, scabies, and viral infections such as the common cold are all _____.

9. Syphilis is a type of _____.

10. Parasites cannot live without a _____.

11. Molds, mildews, and yeasts are all types of _____.

12. The skin disease caused by the itch mite is _____.

13. _____ immunity is partly inherited.

14. When the body overcomes a disease, it develops _____ immunity.

15. Acquired immunity can be developed through _____.

TOPIC 2: PRINCIPLES OF PREVENTION

1. The federal agency that enforces safety and health standards in the workplace is _____ _____.

2. The Occupational Safety and Health Act of 1970 regulates employee exposure to _____ substances.

3. Most objects or surfaces in your surroundings are _____, which means they have microorganisms in or on them.

4. The three main levels of decontamination are:

   a) _____

   b) _____

   c) _____

5. _____ kills all microorganisms, including bacterial spores.

6. An autoclave sterilizes tools by the use of _____ under pressure.

7. Disinfection kills most microorganisms on hard, _____ surfaces.

8. Disinfection does not kill _____.

9. _____ should not be used on human skin, hair, or nails.

10. All disinfectants must be approved by the federal agency called the _____ _____.

11. Manufacturers are required to provide information about their products in a _____ _____.

12. A disinfectant that is effective against the *Pseudomonas* bacteria is called _____.

13. Any implement that comes into contact with blood or body fluids must be disinfected in an EPA-registered tuberculocidal disinfectant or a disinfectant that kills _____ and _____.

14. Which disinfectants have the following characteristics?

   a) _____ not a legal disinfectant in most states

   b) _____ nontoxic, odorless, and fast-acting

   c) _____ effective laundry additive

   d) _____ caustic poison

15. You should always wear _____ and _____ when mixing disinfectants.

16. An important rule when mixing disinfectants is to add _____ to _____ .

17. The purpose of wet sanitizers is to _____ .

18. Any item used on a client must be _____ or _____ .

19. If unwashed, damp linens are left in a laundry cart, _____ or _____ may grow on them and on the cart.

20. Touching an object, such as the skin, and then touching another object or product with the same hand or utensil results in _____ .

21. _____ supplies and implements are thrown away after use.

22. Products used in skin care treatments should be removed from their containers with a _____ _____ .

23. Once you have begun a salon treatment, do not open any package or container without a spatula or _____ .

24. It is particularly important to wear gloves during and after:

   a) _____

   b) _____

   c) _____

25. The lowest level of decontamination is _____ .

26. _____ may kill bacteria or prevent their growth, but they are not classified as disinfectants.

27. Showers and other wet rooms should be built with _____ that remove steam.

28. Lancets and other tools that puncture the skin must be decontaminated by dry heat or in a _____ _____ .

29. Nonporous tools such as tweezers, scissors, and plastic spatulas that have not come in contact with blood should be decontaminated by complete immersion in an EPA-registered, hospital-grade disinfectant that is:

    a) _____

    b) _____

    c) _____

    d) _____

30. Universal Precautions require that employers and employees assume that all human _____ and _____ are infectious for HIV, HBV, and other bloodborne pathogens.

RAPID REVIEW TEST

Date: _____

Rating: _____

Insert the correct term in the space provided.

aseptic	dry heat	pathogens
asymptomatic	efficacy	sodium hypochlorite
contaminants	formalin	sterilized
decontamination	glass electrodes	styptic
double-bagging	immersion	Universal Precautions

1. Dirt, oils, makeup on a brush, or lotion on a cotton pad are all _____ .

2. Removing, inactivating, or destroying pathogens is called _____ .

3. Methods of sterilization include the autoclave and _____ .

4. Tools that come into contact with blood or other bodily fluids must be _____ .

5. Items such as _____ cannot be sterilized in an autoclave because they will break.

6. Any disinfectant used in a salon must have the correct _____ , or effectiveness against pathogens.

7. _____ was used as a disinfectant in the past but is no longer considered safe for salon use.

8. The chemical term for household bleach is _____.

9. Proper disinfection procedure requires complete _____ in disinfectant for the required amount of time.

10. Handling sterilized and disinfected equipment and supplies so they are not contaminated until they are used on a client is called _____ procedure.

11. In a blood spill, after cleaning the wound, apply antiseptic or _____.

12. Contaminated disposable objects such as cotton balls should be discarded by _____.

13. To sanitize is to significantly reduce the number of _____ on a surface.

14. OSHA prescribes the use of _____ as the approach to infection control.

15. A client who is _____ shows no symptoms or signs of infection.

4

ANATOMY AND PHYSIOLOGY

Date: _____

Rating: _____

Text pages: 58–95

TOPIC 1: CELLS

1. The study of the functions and activities performed by the body structures is _____ .

2. The study of body structures that can be seen with the naked eye, and what they are made up of, is _____ .

3. _____ is the science of the minute structures of organic tissues.

4. What is a cell? _____

5. Describe protoplasm. _____
   _____

6. Match the following cell structures to their definitions:

   cell membrane   cytoplasm   nucleus

   a) _____   all the protoplasm of a cell except that which is in the nucleus

   b) _____   structure that encloses the protoplasm

   c) _____   dense protoplasm found in the center of the cell

7. Cells divide into two identical cells called _____ .

8. Constructive metabolism, in which larger molecules are built from smaller ones, is called _____
   _____ .

9. The phase of metabolism in which complex compounds are broken down into smaller ones is called
   _____ .

10. Body tissues are composed of 60 to 90 percent _____ .

11. Match each of these examples of tissue with its tissue type:

bone   muscle   spinal cord
lymph   skin

a) _____   muscular tissue

b) _____   connective tissue

c) _____   liquid tissue

d) _____   nerve tissue

e) _____   epithelial tissue

12. Match each of these organs with its function:

heart   lungs   stomach
kidneys   liver

a) _____   supply oxygen to the blood

b) _____   removes toxic products of digestion

c) _____   excrete water and waste products

d) _____   digests food

e) _____   circulates the blood

13. List the ten major body systems:

a) _____

b) _____

c) _____

d) _____

e) _____

f) _____

g) _____

h) _____

i) _____

j) _____

RAPID REVIEW TEST

Date: _____

Rating: _____

Insert the correct term in the space provided.

epithelial tissue   metabolism   organ

glands   mitosis   system

liquid tissue   nervous system

1. Most cells reproduce in a process known as _____.

2. Anabolism and catabolism are the two phases of _____.

3. The tissue that carries food, hormones, and waste products through the body is _____.

4. _____ is the tissue that supports, protects, and binds together other body tissues.

5. A/an _____ is a group of tissues that perform a specific function.

6. A _____ is made up of organs working together to perform one or more functions.

7. The endocrine system is made up of specialized _____.

8. The brain and spinal cord are part of the _____.

TOPIC 2: THE SKELETAL SYSTEM

1. How many bones are there in the skeletal system? _____

2. Bones are connected by movable and immovable _____.

3. Bone is composed of about two-thirds _____ matter.

4. Name the five primary functions of the skeletal system:

   a) _____

   b) _____

   c) _____

   d) _____

   e) _____

5. Elbows and knees are examples of _____ joints.

6. The skull is divided into two parts, the _____ and the _____ .

7. Use the following two illustrations to identify the bones of the cranium and face in the corresponding spaces.

a) _____

b _____

c) _____

d) _____

e) _____

f) _____

g) _____

h) _____

i) _____

j) _____

k) _____

8. Match these cranial bones with their descriptions:

ethmoid bone   occipital bone   sphenoid bone

frontal bone   parietal bones   temporal bones

a) _____ joins all the bones of the cranium together

b) _____ forms the forehead

c) _____ hindmost bone of the skull

d) _____ form the sides of the head in the ear region

e) _____ form the sides and crown of the cranium

f) _____ bone between the eye sockets

9. Identify the bones of the neck, shoulder, and back in the corresponding spaces.

a) _____

b) _____

c) _____

d) _____

e) _____

f) _____

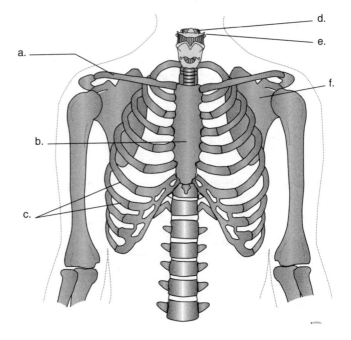

10. The _____ is a U-shaped bone at the base of the tongue.

11. How many pairs of ribs are there in the thorax? _____

12. Match these bones of the shoulder, arm, and hand with their definitions:

carpus   clavicle   humerus
metacarpus   phalanges   radius
scapula   ulna

a) _____ shoulder blade

b) _____ palm

c) _____ collarbone

d) _____ larger bone of the forearm

e) _____ largest bone of the arm

f) _____ finger bones

g) _____ wrist

h) _____ smaller bone of the forearm

13. Each shoulder consists of one _____ and one

_____ .

14. The thorax protects the heart, _____ , and other internal organs.

15. Identify the bones of the arm in the corresponding spaces.

a) _____

b) _____

c) _____

d) _____

RAPID REVIEW TEST

Date: _____

Rating: _____

Insert the correct term in the space provided.

Adam's apple	lacrimal bones	radius
cervical vertebrae	lower jawbone	sternum
cheekbones	maxillae	

1. The bones of the upper jaw are the _____.

2. The mandible forms the _____.

3. The eye sockets are formed by small, thin bones called the _____.

4. The two zygomatic or malar bones form the _____.

5. The hyoid bone is also called the _____.

6. Part of the thorax is the _____ or breastbone.

7. The smaller forearm bone, on the thumb side, is the _____.

8. The uppermost seven bones of the vertebral column are called the _____.

TOPIC 3: THE MUSCULAR SYSTEM

1. What are the main functions of the muscular system?

   a) _____

   b) _____

2. The body has over 600 muscles, which account for approximately _____ percent of its weight.

3. What are the three types of muscle tissue?

   a) _____

   b) _____

   c) _____

4. The _____ is the part of the muscle that does not move.

5. The _____ is the part of the muscle at the more movable attachment to the skeleton.

6. Pressure in massage is usually directed from the _____ to the _____ .

7. List seven ways in which muscular tissue can be stimulated.

a) _____   e) _____

b) _____   f) _____

c) _____   g) _____

d) _____

8. The following muscles are located in the scalp, neck, ear, eyebrow, nose, and mouth. Indicate where each of these muscles is located.

a) _____   orbicularis oris

b) _____   orbicularis oculi

c) _____   frontalis

d) _____   auricularis anterior

e) _____   procerus

f) _____   sternocleidomastoideus

9. Identify the muscles of the head, face, and neck in the corresponding spaces.

a) _____

b) _____

c) _____

d) _____

e) _____

f) _____

g) _____

h) _____

i) _____

j) _____

k) _____

l) _____

m) _____

n) _____

o) _____

p) _____

10. The _____ is the broad muscle that covers the top of the skull.

11. The _____ superior, anterior, and posterior are the muscles of the ear.

12. The masseter and temporalis muscles are sometimes referred to as the _____ muscles.

13. The eyebrow muscle that draws the eyebrow down and wrinkles the forehead vertically is the _____ _____ muscle.

14. The _____ covers the bridge of the nose and lowers the eyebrows.

15. Match each of these muscles to its function:

buccinator   levator labii superioris   risorius
depressor labii inferioris   mentalis   triangularis
levator anguli oris   orbicularis oris   zygomaticus major/minor

a) _____ compresses the cheeks and expels air between the lips

b) _____ draws the corner of the mouth out and back, as in grinning

c) _____ compresses, contracts, puckers, and wrinkles the lips

d) _____ raises the angle of the mouth and draws it inward

e) _____ elevates the lower lip and raises and wrinkles the skin of the chin

f) _____ depresses the lower lip and draws it to one side

g) _____ elevates the lip, as in laughing

h) _____ elevates the upper lip and dilates the nostrils, as in expressing distaste

i) _____ pulls down the corners of the mouth

16. The broad, flat muscle covering the back of the neck and upper and middle region of the back controling the shoulder blade is the _____ .

17. The _____ is a muscle of the chest that assists in breathing and in raising the arm.

18. Match each of these muscles in the shoulder or arm to its description:

biceps   flexors   supinator
deltoid   pronators   triceps
extensors

a) _____   wrist muscles involved in bending the wrist

b) _____   muscle producing the contour of the front and inner side of the upper arm

c) _____   muscles that straighten the wrist, hand, and fingers

d) _____   large muscle that covers the entire back of the upper arm and extends the forearm

e) _____   muscle that rotates the radius outward and the palm upward

f) _____   muscles that turn the hand inward so that the palm faces downward

g) _____   large, triangular muscle covering the shoulder joint

19. Identify the muscles of the shoulder and arm in the corresponding spaces.

a) _____

b) _____

c) _____

d) _____

e) _____

f) _____

g) _____

a.
b.
c.
d.
e.

Anterior or palm

f.
g.
g.

Posterior or back of hand

RAPID REVIEW TEST

Date: _____

Rating: _____

Insert the correct term in the space provided.

aponeurosis   orbicularis oculi   sternocleidomastoideus
heart   pectoralis   striated
nonstriated   platysma   trapezius
occipitalis

1. _____ muscles function automatically, without conscious will.

2. Cardiac muscle is found only in the _____ .

3. The muscles that are attached to the bones and are controlled by the will are _____ muscles.

4. The back of epicranius, called the _____ , draws the scalp backward.

5. The tendon that connects the occipitalis and frontalis is the _____ .

6. The _____ extends from the chest and shoulder muscles to the side of the chin.

7. The _____ lowers and rotates the head.

8. The ring muscle of the eye socket that closes the eye is the _____ .

9. The _____ covers the back of the neck and upper and middle regions of the back and helps to rotate the arm.

10. The _____ major and minor are muscles of the chest that assist the swinging movements of the arm.

TOPIC 4: THE NERVOUS SYSTEM

1. What is the primary function of the nervous system? _____

   _____

2. Name the principal components of the nervous system.

   a) _____

   b) _____

   c) _____

3. What are the three main subdivisions of the nervous system?

   a) _____

   b) _____

   c) _____

4. The spinal cord, spinal nerves, and cranial nerves make up the _____ or

   _____ system.

5. The _____ nervous system controls the involuntary muscles, such as the glands, blood vessels, and heart.

6. The _____ nervous system carries impulses, or messages, to and from the central nervous system.

7. What is the largest, most complex nerve tissue in the body? _____

8. How many pairs of cranial nerves originate in the brain? _____
   How many pairs of spinal nerves extend from the spinal cord? _____

9. Where are the spinal nerves distributed? _____

10. A nerve cell is also called a _____.

11. What is the function of dendrites? _____

    _____

12. What is the function of the axon? _____

    _____

13. Which type of nerve carries impulses from the brain to the muscles? _____

14. Which type of nerve carries impulses from the sense organs to the brain? _____

15. Pulling the hand away quickly from a hot stove is an example of a _____ .

16. The _____ is also known as the trifacial or trigeminal nerve.

17. The three branches of the trifacial or trigeminal nerve are the:

   a) _____

   b) _____

   c) _____

18. Identify the nerves of the head, face, and neck in the corresponding spaces.

   a) _____

   b) _____

   c) _____

   d) _____

   e) _____

   f) _____

   g) _____

   h) _____

   i) _____

   j) _____

   k) _____

   l) _____

   m) _____

   n) _____

   o) _____

   p) _____

   q) _____

   r) _____

19. Match each of the following nerves with its function:

auriculotemporal	mental	supratrochlear
infraorbital	nasal	zygomatic
infratrochlear	supraorbital	

a) _____ affects the skin of the lower eyelid, side of the nose, upper lip, and mouth

b) _____ affects the skin between the eyes and upper side of the nose

c) _____ affects the skin of the lower lip and chin

d) _____ affects the external ear and skin above the temple, up to the top of the skull

e) _____ affects the muscles of the upper part of the cheek

f) _____ affects the membrane and skin of the nose

g) _____ affects the skin of the forehead, scalp, eyebrow, and upper eyelid

h) _____ affects the point and lower side of the nose

20. The chief motor nerve of the face is the _____ nerve.

21. Match each of the following nerves with its function:

| buccal | posterior auricular | temporal |
| cervical | mandibular | zygomatic |

a) _____ affects the muscles of the temple, side of the forehead, eyebrow, eyelid, and upper part of the cheek

b) _____ affects the side of the neck and the platysma muscle

c) _____ affects the muscles of the lower lip and chin

d) _____ affects the muscles of the mouth

e) _____ affects the muscles of the upper part of the cheek

f) _____ affects the muscles behind the ear at the base of the skull

22. Match each of the following cervical nerves with its function:

       cervical cutaneous   greater occipital

       greater auricular   smaller occipital

a) _____ affects the scalp and muscles behind the ear

b) _____ affects the face, ears, neck, and parotid gland

c) _____ affects the scalp as far up as the top of the head

d) _____ affects the front and sides of the neck as far down as the breastbone

23. List the principal nerves of the arm and hand and what parts they supply.

a) _____

b) _____

c) _____

d) _____

TOPIC 5: THE CIRCULATORY SYSTEM

1. What is the primary function of the circulatory system? _____

_____

2. Name the two divisions of the circulatory system and their components:

a) _____

b) _____

3. What is the function of lymph? _____

4. What is the function of the heart? _____

5. Identify the parts of the heart in the corresponding spaces.

a) _____

b) _____

c) _____

d) _____

e) _____

f) _____

g) _____

h) _____

i) _____

j) _____

k) _____

l) _____

6. The interior of the heart contains four chambers and _____ valves.

7. When the heart contracts and relaxes, blood flows in, then travels from the _____ to the _____ and out of the heart.

8. What is the normal heartbeat rate in a resting state? _____

9. Name the functions of the following:

a) pulmonary circulation _____

b) systemic circulation _____

c) arteries _____

d) capillaries _____
_____

e) veins _____

10. Blood has the following characteristics:

a) There are _____ pints in the human body.

b) Blood is about _____ percent water.

c) The normal temperature of blood is _____ Fahrenheit.

d) Blood is bright red in the _____ and dark red in the _____ .

e) Blood is composed of red and white _____ , _____ ,
_____ , and _____ .

11. Name the five primary functions of blood.

a) _____

b) _____
_____

c) _____

d) _____
_____

e) _____

12. Red blood cells or corpuscles are produced in the _____ .

13. Name the functions of these components of blood:

a) red blood cells   _____

b) white blood cells   _____

c) platelets   _____

d) plasma   _____
_____

14. Lymph is filtered by lymph nodes, a process that helps fight _____ .

15. Name the four primary functions of lymph.

a) _____

b) _____

c) _____

d) _____

16. Identify the arteries of the head, face, and neck in the corresponding spaces.

a) _____

b) _____

c) _____

d) _____

e) _____

f) _____

g) _____

h) _____

i) _____

j) _____

k) _____

l) _____

m) _____

n) _____

o) _____

p) _____

17. The main source of blood supply to the head, face, and neck is the _____ arteries.

18. Match each of the following arteries with the area to which it supplies blood.

angular artery   middle temporal artery   submental artery

anterior auricular artery   occipital artery   superior labial artery

frontal artery   parietal artery   supraorbital artery

inferior labial artery   posterior auricular artery   transverse facial artery

infraorbital artery

a) _____ forehead and upper eyelids

b) _____ scalp, the area behind and above the ear, and the skin behind the ear

c) _____ upper eyelid and forehead

d) _____ upper lip and region of the nose

e) _____   side of the nose

f) _____   muscles of the eye

g) _____   temples

h) _____   chin and lower lip

i) _____   skin and masseter

j) _____   front part of the ear

k) _____   skin and muscles of the scalp and back of the head up to the crown

l) _____   side and crown of the head

m) _____   lower lip

19. The two principal veins on each side of the neck are the internal and external _____.

20. _____ are found deep in the tissues, while _____ are closer to the surface of the arms and hands.

RAPID REVIEW TEST

Date: _____

Rating: _____

Insert the correct term in the space provided.

aorta   leukocytes   ulnar
atrium   pericardium   valve
erythrocytes   platelets   ventricle
hemoglobin   radial

1. The heart is enclosed by a membrane called the _____.

2. The upper, thin-walled chambers of the heart are the right and left _____.

3. A _____ is one of the lower, thick-walled chambers of the heart.

4. A _____ is a structure between the chambers of the heart that allows blood to flow in only one direction.

5. The largest artery in the body is the _____.

6. Red blood cells are also called _____.

7. _____ is the iron protein that gives blood its bright red color.

8. White blood cells are also called _____.

9. Thrombocytes are also called _____.

10. The _____ artery and its branches supply the little finger side of the arm and palm of the hand.

11. The _____ artery and its branches supply the thumb side of the arm and the back of the hand.

TOPIC 6: OTHER BODY SYSTEMS

1. The _____ system comprises glands that affect the growth, development, sexual activities, and health of the body.

2. Specialized organs that remove certain elements from the blood and convert them into new compounds are called _____.

3. What is the difference between exocrine and endocrine glands? _____

_____

_____

4. Sweat and oil glands are types of _____ glands.

5. Insulin, adrenaline, and estrogen are _____.

6. Digestive _____ are chemicals that change certain kinds of food into a form that can be used by the body.

7. The entire digestive process takes about _____ hours to complete.

8. The _____ system purifies the body by eliminating waste matter.

9. What does each of the following organs excrete?

   a) skin _____

   b) large intestine _____

   c) kidneys _____

   d) liver _____

   e) lungs _____

10. The respiratory system consists of the _____ and air passages.

11. During inhalation, _____ is absorbed into the blood.

12. During exhalation, the lungs expel _____.

13. The respiratory system is protected on both sides by the _____.

14. The muscular wall that separates the thorax from the abdominal region is the _____.

5

CHEMISTRY FOR ESTHETICIANS

Date: _____

Rating: _____

Text pages: 96–113

TOPIC 1: BRANCHES OF CHEMISTRY

1. Why is it important for estheticians to have a basic knowledge of chemistry?

   a) _____

   b) _____

2. Define *chemistry*. _is the science that deals with the Composition, Structure, and Properties of matter._

3. The two branches of chemistry are _Organic_ and _Inorganic_ .

4. Organic chemistry studies substances that contain _Carbon_ .

5. Gasoline, plastics, synthetic fabrics, pesticides, and fertilizers are manufactured from natural gas and oil and are therefore considered _Organic_ .

6. Metals, minerals, pure water, and clean air do not burn and are considered _Inorganic_ .

TOPIC 2: MATTER

1. Define *matter*. _is any substance that occupies space, has physical & chemical Properties, and exists in the form of a Solid, liquid or gas._

2. List the three states of matter, their primary characteristics, and an example of each.

   a) _Solid have a definite shape and Volume. Ice is an Example of a Solid_

   b) _Liquids have a definite Volume but not a definite shape; they take the shape Containers. Water is an example of a liquid_

   c) _Gases do not have a definite Volume or shape. They expand easily and Can be Compressed Steam is an example of a gas._

3. What is an element? _is the basic unit of all matter_

4. How many naturally occurring elements are there? _90_

5. Elements are made up of structural units called _Atoms_.

6. Name the smaller particles that make up atoms and the electrical charge of each:

   a) _protons, which have a positive electrical charge_

   b) _neutrons, with a neutral charge;_

   c) _electrons, with a negative charge_

7. Joining two or more atoms chemically creates a _____.

8. Elemental molecules contain two or more atoms of the same element that are united _chemically_.

9. Chemical combinations of two or more atoms of different elements are _Compound molecules_.

10. Define *compound*. _is a Combination of two or more atoms of different elements_

11. What is the chemical composition of water? _H_2O_

12. Define *mixture*. _is a Combination of two or more substances united physically, not chemically, without a fixed composition and in any proportion._

13. Color, weight, melting point, and odor are examples of _Physical_ properties.

14. When wood is burned and turns into ash, there is a change in its _chemical_ properties.

15. Define these terms and give an example of each:

   a) physical change: _is a change in the form or physical properties of a substance without the formation of a new substance, solid ice undergoes a physical_

   b) chemical change: _is a change in the chemical composition of a substance_

16. Identify the following elements, compounds, or mixtures in the spaces provided:

a) _Air_   gaseous mixture that makes up the earth's atmosphere

b) _Oxygen_   most abundant element found both free and in compounds

c) _Hydrogen peroxide_   colorless liquid that is a compound of hydrogen and oxygen

d) _Nitrogen_   gaseous element that comprises about four-fifths of the air

e) _Water_   most abundant of all substances; comprising about 75 percent of the earth's surface

f) _hydrogen_   lightest element known; flammable and explosive when mixed with air

17. Oxygen combines with many other elements to form compounds called _oxides_.

18. _Nitrogen_ is found mostly in the form of ammonia and nitrates.

19. One of the important chemical characteristics of oxygen is its ability to support _Combustion_.

20. The most commonly used ingredient in cosmetics is _Water_.

21. A 10 percent volume solution of _____ has antiseptic properties.

22. What is pH? _____

23. Name the characteristics of acids and alkalis/bases:

a) acids: _____

b) alkalis or bases: _____

24. What is the neutral pH range? _7.0_

25. A pH of 6 is _____ times more alkaline than a pH of 5, and _____ times more alkaline than a pH of 4.

26. What are the functions of the acid mantle? _is a protective barrier again certain forms of bacteria and microorganisms, and it may be a factor in the natural skin shedding and renewal process._

27. What is the pH of the acid mantle? _between 4.5 and 6.2_

28. _Inflammation_ may result if the skin is exposed to low or high pH.

29. When equal proportions of an acid and an alkali are combined, they neutralize each other and form ____ _H_2O_ and a salt.

30. Define the following terms:

    a) oxidation: _is a chemical reaction that combines an element or compound with oxygen to produce an oxide._

    b) reduction: _when oxygen is subtracted from a substance, the substance is reduced_

    c) combustion: _is the rapid oxidation of any substance_

    d) redox: _is a contraction for reduction oxidation_

31. An oxidizing agent releases _____ .

32. Oxidation and _____ always occur at the same time.

33. Solutions, suspensions, and emulsions are all kinds of _____ .

34. Identify the following substances in the spaces provided:

    a) _Solvent._ substance, usually liquid, that dissolves another substance to form a solution, with no change in chemical composition

    b) _Suspension_ state in which solid particles are distributed throughout a liquid medium

    c) _Solution_ blended mixture of two or more solids, liquids, or gaseous substances

    d) _emulsion_ mixture of two or more immiscible substances united with the aid of a binder or emulsifier

    e) _____ the dissolved substance in a solution

    f) _Miscible_ liquids that are mutually soluble; can be mixed with each other in any proportion without separating

35. _Water_ is a universal solvent.

36. Define *immiscible liquids* and give an example. _are not Capable of being Mixed. Water and oil are immiscible liquids_

37. List three characteristics of solutions:

     a) _____

     b) _____

     c) _____

38. List three characteristics of suspensions:

     a) _____

        _____

     b) _____

     c) _____

39. What does the term *emulsify* mean? _to form an emulsion_

40. What are the substances that allow oil and water to mix? _Molecule_

41. Name and describe the two parts of a surfactant molecule.

     a) _The head of the surfactant molecule is hydrophilic, meaning water-loving._

     b) _The tail is lipophilic, meaning oil-loving_

42. Match each of the following substances with the type of matter it represents.

     compound   emulsion   suspension

     element   solution

     a) _____ pure water

     b) _____ salt water

     c) _____ carbon

     d) _Compound_ shampoo

     e) _emulsion_ calamine lotion

43. List and define the two types of emulsions used in cosmetics.

a) _____

b) _____

44. O/W emulsions usually contain more _____ than _____.

45. What is one advantage of O/W emulsions? _____

46. Give examples of O/W emulsions. _____

47. Give examples of W/O emulsions. _____

_____

48. If a cosmetic emulsion product separates, it should be _____.

COSMETIC CHEMISTRY

Date: _____

Rating: _____

Text pages: 114–131

TOPIC 1: COSMETIC INGREDIENTS

1. The FDA views cosmetics in accordance with the _____ of 1938.

2. How are cosmetics defined by the FDA? _____
   _____
   _____

3. According to the FDA, how are drugs different from cosmetics? _____
   _____

4. Estheticians focus on improving the skin's appearance. They cannot claim that a product or treatment
   _____ .

5. Name and describe the two basic types of cosmetic ingredients.

   a) _____
   _____

   b) _____

6. What other terms are used to refer to performance ingredients?

   a) _____

   b) _____

   c) _____

7. What is the action of each of these ingredients on the skin?

   a) alphahydroxy acids _____

   b) glycerin _____

   c) lipids _____

8. _____ are products intended to improve the skin's health and appearance.

9. What are the functions of water in cosmetics?

   a) as a vehicle: _____

   b) as a performance ingredient: _____

10. Almost all skin care products are a mixture of _____ and _____ .

11. Anhydrous products are generally designed for _____ skin.

12. Emollients are almost always _____ agents.

13. Emollients lie on top of the skin and prevent _____ by trapping water, a process called _____ .

14. Name five advantages of mineral oil and petrolatum in cosmetic formulations.

   a) _____

   b) _____

   c) _____

   d) _____

   e) _____

15. Why do mineral oil and petrolatum not need preservatives? _____
    _____

16. Plant oils are very similar to human _____ , which is beneficial for skin that does not produce enough.

17. Identify these emollients in the spaces provided:

   a) _____ lubricant ingredients derived from plant oils or animal fats

   b) _____ mineral-based substances used as lightweight emollients and vehicles

   c) _____ emollients produced from fatty acids and alcohols

   d) _____ fatty acids that have been exposed to hydrogen

18. List the benefits of the following emollient ingredients:

   a) fatty esters: _____

   b) fatty acids: _____

   c) fatty alcohols: _____

   d) silicones: _____

   _____

19. Emollients that block the pores are said to be _____ .

20. _____ are ingredients that reduce the surface tension between the skin and the product.

21. Comedogenic products should not be used on clog-prone or _____ skin.

22. The main surfactant used in skin care products is _____ .

23. Without _____ , the oil and water in a product would separate into layers.

24. Substances that are compatible with oil and mixed into the oil phase of a product are called _____

   _____ .

25. _____ are nonfoaming, oil-in-water emulsions that are excellent for removing makeup.

26. What are aromatherapy or essential oils? _____

   _____

27. What are the two functions of preservatives in cosmetic products?

   a) _____

   _____

   b) _____

28. What are antioxidants? _____

   _____

29. The government agency that regulates color agents in cosmetics is the _____ .

30. Name and describe the two types of color ingredients.

a) _____

_____

_____

b) _____

_____

_____

31. Hydrators, or humectants, attract _____ to the skin's surface.

32. Most moisturizing products are combinations of _____ and _____ .

33. _____ is the removal of dead corneum cells.

34. How do mechanical exfoliating ingredients work on the skin? _____

_____

35. How do chemical exfoliating ingredients work? _____

_____

36. What are the three ways in which delivery systems are used?

a) _____

b) _____

c) _____

37. Name two commonly used delivery systems.

a) _____

b) _____

38. Advanced skin care treatments can help the skin function at maximum capacity at any age and slow the appearance of _____ .

39. Name four high-tech antioxidants that stimulate metabolic processes and describe briefly how they help the skin.

a) _____

_____

_____

b) _____

c) _____

_____

d) _____

_____

_____

40. What are the two general categories of masks, and what is the main difference between them?

a) _____

b) _____

41. Name the three basic functions of setting masks.

a) _____

b) _____

c) _____

42. Setting masks generally use _____ as their base.

43. Nonsetting masks are intended mostly for _____ and sensitive skins.

44. _____ or concentrates are designed as a corrective treatment to be used for 30 to 60 days or more.

45. Professional _____ are corrective treatments intended for immediate, one-time use.

46. The OTC drug product most commonly used by estheticians is _____ .

47. Sunscreens either _____ or _____ the sun's ultraviolet rays.

48. Name and briefly describe the two types of sunscreens.

a) _____

b) _____

RAPID REVIEW TEST

Date: _____

Rating: _____

Insert the correct term in the space provided.

anhydrous   comedogenicity   liposomes
broad-spectrum   delivery systems   mechanical exfoliating
carbomers   detergents   ingredients
chemical exfoliating ingredients   emollients   physical or particulate sunscreens
cleansing milks   emulsifier   polymers
cold cream   hydrators   serums
comedogenic   inert   yeast cells

1. _____ products do not contain any water.

2. When used as vehicles, _____ place, spread, and keep other agents on the skin.

3. Mineral oil and petrolatum are nonreactive and biologically _____.

4. One of the earliest moisturizers was _____.

5. Safflower, sunflower, and canola oil are lighter and less _____ than coconut oil and palm oil.

6. The tendency of a topical product to cause or worsen a build-up of dead cells in the follicles that leads to development of a blackhead is called _____.

7. The ingredients that cause cleansers to foam are _____.

8. Oils and water are blended in a product with the aid of an _____.

9. Emulsion cleansers are commonly known as _____.

10. _____ are used to thicken cream and gel products.

11. Glycerin, seaweed extracts, and algae extract are types of _____ or humectants.

12. Alphahydroxy acids, betahydroxy acids, and enzymes are examples of _____
_____.

13. Jojoba beads and ground almonds are types of _____.

14. The chemical techniques that use vehicles to make products work are called _____.

15. _____ are vehicles that deliver ingredients to the skin by dissolving them over time.

16. _____ , or microsponges, are vehicles that release substances on the skin's surface at a microscopically controlled rate.

17. Polyglucans, beta-glucans, TRF, and glycoproteins are derived from _____.

18. _____ are considered user-friendly versions of ampoules.

19. Zinc oxide or titanium oxide is the functional ingredient in _____ sunscreens.

20. Both physical and absorbing sunscreens can be combined into one product to provide _____ protection.

TOPIC 2: MAKEUP INGREDIENTS

1. Oil-based foundation contains _____ oil, while the main ingredient in oil-free foundation is _____.

2. Face powder is made up of a powder base mixed with a _____ and perfume.

3. The two categories of cream and liquid cheek colors are oil-based and _____.

4. _____ or detergents added to cream cheek color allow it to penetrate hair follicles and cracks in the skin.

5. The main ingredient in lipsticks is _____.

6. Stick and cream eye shadows are _____-based, with oil, petrolatum, and other ingredients added.

7. Eyeliner pencils consist of a _____ hardened oil base.

8. The pigments in mascara must be _____ , or unable to combine with other ingredients.

9. Some _____ mascaras contain rayon or nylon fibers.

10. Specialized cosmetics that diminish skin imperfections or skin disfigurements are used in _____ _____ makeup applications.

TOPIC 3: NATURAL INGREDIENTS AND OTHER TOPICS

1. One drawback of natural ingredients is that they may cause _____ in sensitive clients.

2. An ingredient in cosmetic formulations that was originally derived from roosters' combs is _____

   _____ .

3. How can estheticians make informed choices between natural and bioengineered cosmetics?

   _____

4. What are the disadvantages of using homemade products in the salon?

   a) _____

   _____

   b) _____

   c) _____

   _____

5. The FDA regulates cosmetics only in terms of _____ or claims.

6. Only claims related to _____ can be made for cosmetics.

7. According to FDA regulations, product ingredients must be listed in _____ order, from the ingredient with the highest concentration to that with the lowest concentration.

8. Name six possible symptoms of an allergic reaction to a cosmetic ingredient.

   a) _____

   b) _____

   c) _____

   d) _____

   e) _____

   f) _____

9. The best way to avoid an allergic reaction in a client is with a _____ on the arm.

10. Sanitary procedures you should always follow in the salon include:

a) _____

b) _____

c) _____

d) _____

e) _____

7

BASICS OF ELECTRICITY

Date: _____

Rating: _____

Text pages: 132–148

TOPIC 1: ELECTRICITY

1. Define *electricity*. _____

   _____

2. Electricity is a flow of subatomic particles called _____ .

3. An electric current is the flow of electricity along a _____ .

4. A substance that does not easily transmit electricity is called a nonconductor or _____ .

5. In electric wires, the twisted metal threads are the _____ , and the rubber or silk that covers them are _____ .

6. What is the difference between direct and alternating current? _____

   _____

   _____

   _____

7. What is the difference between a converter and a rectifier? _____

   _____

8. What do the following electrical units measure?

   a) volt _____

   b) ohm _____

   c) amp _____

   d) watt _____

9. One-thousandth of an ampere is a _____ .

10. One thousand watts is a _____ .

11. Match each of the following electrical devices to its function:

circuit breaker   milliampere meter   polarity changer
fuse   plug   rheostat
jack

a) _____   switch that reverses with the direction of the current from positive to negative and vice versa

b) _____   prong connector at the end of an electrical cord that connects an apparatus to an electrical outlet

c) _____   device that prevents excessive current from passing through a circuit

d) _____   control that regulates the strength of the current used

e) _____   plug-in device used to make electrical contact

f) _____   switch that automatically interrupts or shuts off an electric circuit at the first indication of overload

g) _____   instrument that measures the rate of flow of an electric current

12. The UL symbol on an electrical appliance, which stands for _____, certifies the safety of the appliance.

13. Electrical plugs with one prong that is slightly larger than the other can only be inserted in one way and protect you from _____ in case of a short circuit.

14. Fill in the missing terms in the following precautions:

a) When appliances are not being used, they should be _____.

b) Use _____ plug(s) per outlet.

c) Avoid contact with _____ and metal surfaces when you are using electricity.

d) Disconnect appliances by pulling on the _____.

e) Allowing an electrical cord to become twisted may cause a _____.

f) Do not clean around electric outlets while equipment is _____.

g) Do not leave any client _____ while connected to an electrical device.

RAPID REVIEW TEST

Date: _____

Rating: _____

Insert the correct term in the space provided.

chemical   conductor   mechanical

circuit breakers   ground   second

complete circuit

1. Copper is an especially good _____ .

2. A _____ is the path of an electric current from the generating source back to its original source.

3. Direct current produces a _____ reaction.

4. Alternating current produces a _____ action.

5. A 60-watt light bulb uses 60 watts of energy per _____ .

6. _____ have largely replaced fuses in modern electric circuits.

7. A third, circular prong on an electric plug provides additional _____ .

TOPIC 2: ELECTROTHERAPY

1. The term for electronic facial treatments is _____ .

2. The various currents used in facial and scalp treatments are called _____ .

3. What is polarity? _____

4. Name and briefly describe the two poles of an electric current.

   a) _____

   b) _____

5. What are the four modalities used in cosmetology?

a) _____

b) _____

c) _____

d) _____

6. Describe the galvanic current. _____

_____

7. List the effects of the positive and negative poles of the galvanic current.

Positive Pole (Anode)   Negative Pole (Cathode)

_____   _____

_____   _____

_____   _____

_____   _____

_____   _____

_____   _____

8. Negative galvanic current should not be used on clients with:

a) _____

b) _____

c) _____

d) _____

9. Match the following terms with their descriptions:

anaphoresis   desincrustation
cataphoresis   iontophoresis

_____ process used to soften and emulsify grease deposits and blackheads in the hair follicles

_____ forcing acidic substances into deeper tissues from the positive toward the negative pole

_____ introducing water-soluble products into the skin with electric current, such as the positive and negative poles of a galvanic machine

_____ forcing liquids into tissues from the negative toward the positive pole

10. What is a faradic current, and how is it used? _____
_____
_____
_____

11. What are the benefits of using faradic current in a facial treatment?

   a) _____

   b) _____

   c) _____

   d) _____

   e) _____

   f) _____

   g) _____

12. Sinusoidal current is similar to _____ current but is less irritating.

13. Faradic and sinusoidal currents should never be used longer than _____ minutes.

14. The Tesla high-frequency current is a _____ current that requires only one _____ .

15. The benefits of the Tesla high-frequency current in skin treatments are:

   a) _____

   b) _____

   c) _____

   d) _____

   e) _____

   f) _____

16. What are the two methods used to apply Tesla high-frequency current?

   a) _____

   b) _____

17. In which method of high-frequency current application does the client hold the electrode? _____

_____

18. How can you prevent sparking when handling an electrode? _____

_____

19. A client being treated with Tesla high-frequency current should avoid any contact with _____ .

20. What kind of skin is particularly suited for indirect high-frequency current application? _____

_____

RAPID REVIEW TEST

Date: _____

Rating: _____

Insert the correct term in the space provided.

active	modalities	Tesla high-frequency
desincrustation	sparking	wall plate

1. A _____ is plugged into an ordinary outlet to produce different types of electric currents.

2. Galvanic and high-frequency currents are examples of _____ .

3. In a treatment with galvanic current, the _____ electrode is the one used on the area to be treated.

4. A process using galvanic current that is used to treat acne, milia, and comedones is _____ .

5. The _____ current is commonly called the violet ray.

6. In the direct surface application of high-frequency current, dabbing the electrode on one spot causes _____ , which helps heal acne and other lesions.

TOPIC 3: LIGHT THERAPY

1. Define light therapy. _____

_____

2. _____ is electromagnetic radiation that we can see.

3. A _____ is the distance between the peaks of two successive waves of electromagnetic radiation.

4. Short wavelengths have a higher _____ than longer wavelengths.

5. Visible light makes up _____ percent of natural sunlight.

6. Ultraviolet rays and infrared rays are forms of electromagnetic radiation that are _____ .

7. Among the visible light rays, _____ has the shortest wavelength and _____ has the longest.

8. Artificial light rays are produced for salon use with _____ .

9. _____ rays, also called cold or actinic rays, make up _____ percent of natural sunlight.

10. Name four characteristics of UV rays.

    a) _____

    b) _____

    c) _____

    d) _____

11. Natural sunlight produces vitamin _____ in the skin.

12. UV rays stimulate the production of _____ in the skin.

13. How many new cases of skin cancer are diagnosed each year? _____ What percent of cancer cases is caused by overexposure to UV radiation? _____

14. UV lamps should be kept at a distance of _____ inches from the client.

15. _____ rays make up 60 percent of natural sunlight.

16. Name three characteristics of infrared rays.

    a) _____

    b) _____

    c) _____

17. White light is called the _____.

18. Blue light should be used on oily skin that is _____.

19. Red light produces the most _____.

20. List the beneficial effects of the following forms of light therapy:
    Ultraviolet light:

    a) _____

    b) _____

    c) _____

    d) _____

    e) _____

    f) _____

    Infrared light:

    a) _____

    b) _____

    c) _____

    d) _____

    e) _____

    f) _____

    White light:

    a) _____

    b) _____

    c) _____

Blue light:

a) _____

b) _____

c) _____

d) _____

e) _____

Red light:

a) _____

b) _____

c) _____

d) _____

8

PHYSIOLOGY AND HISTOLOGY OF THE SKIN

Date: _____

Rating: _____

Text pages: 150–183

INTRODUCTION

1. _Skin histology_ is the study of the structure and composition of the tissue of the skin, and physiology is the study of its _funtions of the skin_.

TOPIC 1: STRUCTURE AND FUNCTION OF THE SKIN

1. Healthy skin has certain characteristics.

   a) What are four signs of a healthy skin?

   1. _moist_
   2. _Soft_
   3. _Smooth_
   4. _acidic_

   b) On which parts of the body is the skin the thickest and the thinnest? _Skin is thicker on the palms of the hand and soles of the feet, it is thinnest on the eyelids._

2. List the six primary functions of the skin?

   a) _protection_
   b) _Sensation_
   c) _heat regulartion_
   d) _Excretion_
   e) _Secretion_
   f) _absorption_

3. What substance helps to lubricate and protect the skin? _Sebum and Melanin_

4. Fingernails and toenails serve to protect the hands and feet. What kind of material composes fingernails and toenails? _Hard Keratin_

5. Each square inch (6.452 cm^2) of skin is made up of _15 feet of Blood vessels, 12 feet of nerves, 650 sweat glands & 100 oil glands_.

WORD REVIEW

corneum	melanin	sebum
dermis	pliability	sensation
epidermis	protection	stratum
keratin 角質素, 角蛋白	sebaceous	tactile

TOPIC 2: HISTOLOGY OF THE SKIN

1. The skin contains two clearly defined divisions, the dermis and the epidermis.

   a) Which division is the outermost layer?   _epidermis_

   b) Which division is the innermost layer?   _dermis._

2. The epidermis is made up of many thin layers.

   a) How many layers are found in the epidermis?   _5_

   b) Name the epidermal layer that best fits each of the following descriptions:

      1. Contains a skin pigment   _Stratum germinativum_

      2. Continually being shed and replaced   _Stratum Corneum_

      3. Consists of transparent cells   _Stratum Lucidum_

      4. Is known as a granular layer   _stratum granulosum_

      5. Is known as the spiny layer   _Stratum Spinosum_

3. The dermis of the skin contains two layers.

   a) Name them.

      1. _The papillar Layer_   2. _The Reticular Layer_

   b) Which dermal layer is directly beneath the epidermis?   _The Dermis._

   c) In which dermal layer are the following structures and fluids found?

      1. Hyaluronic acid _are found between the fibers in the reticular Layer._

      2. Looped capillaries and tactile corpuscles _The papillary Layer_

   d) What two protein fibers are found in the deeper layer of the dermis?

      1. _Collagen_   2. _elastin_

4. a) Where is the subcutaneous layer located?   _Bottom of the reticular_

   b) The composition of this layer consists of _adipose (fat)_

5. Name three types of nerve fibers found in the skin and its primary function.

   a) _Motor nerve fibers_

   b) _Sensory nerve fibers_

   c) _Secretory nerve fibers._

6. a) The skin is indented with natural openings that are called _hair_ follicles with sebaceous (oil) glands and _____ of the sudoriferous (sweat) glands.

   b) What glands produce sweat that has no offensive odor? _eccrine glands_

   c) Odors and _____ cause a biological reaction to potential mates.

7. Approximately what percent of the skin is water? _50 — 70 percent_

8. To what is the pigment color of the skin attributed? _Melanin_

9. The skin functions as an organ of sensation and protection. List five physical sensations that skin reacts to.

   a) _Cold receptor_

   b) _Pain receptor_

   c) _Touch receptor_

   d) _Heat receptor_

   e) _Pressure receptor_

10. What is the general and constant internal temperature of a healthy body? _37° celsius_

11. Match the following definitions. Insert the proper term in the space provided.

   (absorption)   sebaceous ✓   stratum germinativum –
   papillary ✓   stratum corneum –   subcutaneous ✓
   reticular layer ✓

   a) _Stratum germinativum_   epidermal layer containing melanin

   b) _Papillary_   skin layer containing elastic fibers

   c) _Reticular Layer_   fatty tissue of the skin

   d) _Stratum Corneum_   epidermal layer containing keratin

   e) _Subcutaneous_   dermal layer containing tactile corpuscles

   f) _Sebaceous_   glands that secrete protective and lubricating oil

   g) _absorption_   limited substances that may enter the skin by this process

12. a) Cells that produce melanin are called _____*Melanosomes.*_____ .

    b) Pigment granules are located in the _____*basal Layer*_____ of the skin.

13. a) What glands produce sweat that has no offensive odor? _____*ecrine glands*_____

    b) Where on the body will you find a high concentration of these glands?

       1. _____*forehead*_____   3. _____*Soles.*_____

       2. _____*palms*_____

14. Aging of the skin is influenced by many factors.

    a) Name three of these factors below.

       1. _____*Sun Exposure*_____   3. _____*environment*_____

       2. _____*Health Habits*_____

    b) _____*ultraviolet Rays*_____ have the greatest impact on how our skin ages.

WORD REVIEW

absorption	germinativum	protection
adipose	granulosum	reticular
corneum	keratin	sebaceous
corpuscle	lucidum	sebum
cuticle	melanin	secretion
dermis	papillary	sensation
epidermis	perspiration	stratum
excretion	pigment	subcutaneous
Fahrenheit	pliability	sudoriferous

RAPID REVIEW TEST

Date: _____

Rating: _____

Insert the correct term in the space provided.

dermis	eyelids	moist
epidermis	largest	sebum

1. A healthy complexion is soft and _____*moist*_____ .

2. The skin is the _____*Largest*_____ organ in the body.

3. The skin is the thinnest on the _____*eyelids*_____ .

4. The two main divisions of the skin are the _____*epidermis*_____ and the _____*dermis*_____ .

5. A function of _____*Sebum*_____ is to lubricate and protect the skin.

STRUCTURE OF THE SKIN

From the following descriptive list of parts of the skin, identify the numbered parts on the illustration. Insert the proper term in the space provided.

adipose tissue
arrector pili muscle
arteries
capillaries
cold receptor
epidermic scales
hair shaft

heat receptor
pain receptor
papilla
papillary layer
pressure receptor
reticular layer
sebaceous duct and gland

stratum germinativum
sudoriferous duct
sudoriferous gland
sweat pore
touch receptor
veins

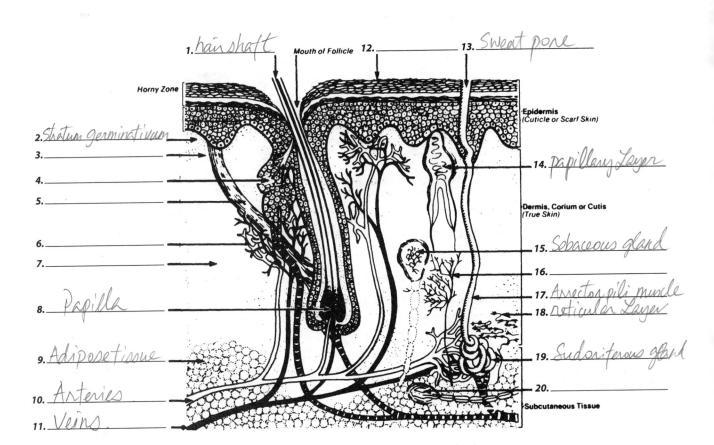

1. *hair shaft*   Mouth of Follicle   12. _____   13. *Sweat pore*

Horny Zone

Epidermis
(Cuticle or Scarf Skin)

2. *Stratum germinativum*

3. _____

4. _____

5. _____

14. *Papillary Layer*

Dermis, Corium or Cutis
(True Skin)

6. _____

7. _____

15. *Sebaceous gland*

16. _____

17. *Arrector pili muscle*

8. *Papilla*

18. *reticular Layer*

9. *Adipose tissue*

19. *Sudoriferous gland*

10. *Arteries*

20. _____

11. *Veins*

Subcutaneous Tissue

TOPIC 3: NUTRITION AND THE HEALTH OF THE SKIN

1. Nutrition is the process by which food is assimilated and converted into tissue in living organisms. Healthy skin is dependent upon good nutrition.

   a) Which two body systems nourish the skin? _The blood & Lymph_

   b) How are the nutrients supplied to the skin? _____

2. The three energy-yielding nutrients include fats, carbohydrates, and proteins.

   a) Why are some fats important to the body? _Some fat is required in diet, essential Component of good health_

   b) What is the most important carbohydrate? _Glucose_

   c) Why is glucose important to the body? _because it provides most of the body's energy._

   d) Are sugars and starches proteins or carbohydrates? _Yes_

   e) What are the chief components of protein? _Muscle tissue, Blood, enzymes._

   f) Which foods are the main sources of protein? (List at least four) _animal meats, fish, eggs, dairy products_

3. Energy is measured in terms of heat units.

   a) What are calories? _Calories fuel the body by making energy_

   b) What happens to calories that are not used by the body? _the body stores the excess Calories as body-fat_

   c) Give an example of a monosaccharide. _____

   d) Starch is classified as a _____.

   e) Why are small amounts of cholesterol needed by the body? _as it is important for cell membranes_

   f) An elevated cholesterol level may be present if a client has _yellow or white papules around the eyes._

4. Minerals are required in the structural composition of hard and soft body tissues. Match the correct name of the mineral with the sentence that best describes its function.

   calcium /   phosphorus   magnesium /
   iron /   potassium /   sodium /

   a) ___Calcium___   critical for development and maintenance of bones and teeth

   b) ___Magnesium___   required for energy release

   c) ___Sodium___   important to the energy metabolism of the cells

d) _Potassium_   required for energy use and water balance

e) _phosphorus_   regulates extracellular fluids. Excessive ingestion can lead to edema

f) _iron_   transports oxygen to cells and is a component of red blood cells

5. When vitamins are listed on a label of food, what do the letters "RDA" mean? _____
Recommended dietary allowances

6. A balanced diet is essential to the health of the entire body and particularly the skin. All vitamins are utilized by the body, but some vitamins are more essential than others for different parts of the body. Match the proper vitamin with the phrase that best describes its importance.

vitamins A   D   K   B2   B6   B1   E   C

a) _A_   Severe deficiency of this vitamin may cause night blindness and skin problems.

b) _B1_   Important for a healthy nervous system and the skin. Helps to prevent beriberi.

c) _K_   Important to the clotting of blood.

d) _B2_   Required in energy production by cells. Deficiency can cause cheilosis.

e) _C_   Required for collagen formation. A lack of this vitamin may lead to poor skin, scurvy, and slow healing.

f) _Vitamin D_   Helps to develop and maintain healthy teeth and bones.

g) _E_   Protects body from damage caused by free radicals.

h) _B6_   Connected with protein synthesis, aids in PMS relief.

7. Vitamins are more abundant in some foods than in others. List two or more natural foods that contain an abundance of the following vitamins.

a) Vitamin A   _Carrots, cheese, tomato_

b) Vitamin B1   _ham & Pork products, oranges._

c) Vitamin C   _Citrus fruit, brussels sprouts, Cauliflower._

d) Vitamin D   _Egg yorks, butterfat, milk._

e) Vitamin E   _Vegetable oils, nuts, meats_

f) Vitamin K   _Liver, Cabbage, green Leaf Vegetable._

g) Folic Acid   _Whole wheat, yeast, dried legumes._

WORD REVIEW

absorption	environment	nutrients
amino acids	enzymes	nutrition
anemia	esophagus	organisms
assimilate	fats	pancreas
balanced diet	food groups	peptide (end bonds)
beriberi	food labels	polypeptides
body processes	gastric juice	protein
calories	glucose	RDA
capillaries	inorganic minerals	salivary glands
carbohydrates	liver	scurvy
circulatory system	lymphatic system	sebum
cholesterol	malnutrition	starch
collagen	metabolism	stomach
connective tissue	minerals	toxic effects
deficiency	molecules	toxicity
dehydration	night blindness	vitamins

TOPIC 4: NUTRITION AND ENVIRONMENT—EFFECTS ON THE SKIN

1. a) The use of tobacco can cause damage to the body inside and out. Name three harmful effects of tobacco use to the skin and body functions.

    1. _____

    2. _____

    3. _____

    b) How does the excessive intake of alcohol affect the skin? (List two) _____

    _____

    c) What is the appearance of dehydrated skin? _____

    _____

2. Water may not be thought of as an element of nutrition, but it is essential to the health of the skin and to efficient functioning of the entire body.

    a) Approximately how much of the body is made up of water? _____ 60% _____

    b) Name at least four ways water helps to keep the body healthy.

    1. _____

    2. _____

3. _____

4. _____

3. The professional esthetician is concerned with the client's total health, but the main concern is the study of nutrition and its effects on the skin.

   a) Why is a well-balanced diet essential to the health and beauty of the skin? _____

   _____

   b) What problems of the skin may be an indication of extremely low-fat diet? _____

   _____

   c) Pellagra is a skin disease characterized by a skin rash. What dietary lack is associated with pellagra? _____

   _____

4. a) Proper nutrition is essential for both physical and mental health. What is the best way to ensure a balance of nutrients? _____

   _____

   b) What must occur in order to lose weight? _____

   _____

WORD REVIEW

alcohol	drugs	scurvy
anemia	estrogen	skin
allergies	jaundice	symptoms
calorie	lesions	temperature
chemical imbalance	malnutrition	tobacco
cholesterol	mental health	vitamin deficiency
dehydrate	nutrition	water
dermatitis	pellagra	

_____

_____

_____

_____

ACTIVITY

Chart everything you eat or drink for two weeks. Using the food pyramid (Figure 8–12 in text, page 167) of the recommended daily allowances, categorize your intake with the food groups and recommended servings per day.

Do you feel your eating habits are those conducive to healthy mind and body?

Did you drink enough water for proper hydration?

Where do you need to increase (or decrease) portions to stay within the pyramid?

How would you adjust your diet to gain weight?

How would you adjust your diet to lose weight?

9

SKIN DISORDERS AND DISEASES

Date: _____

Rating: _____

Text Pages: 184–205

TOPIC 1: UNDERSTANDING SKIN DISORDERS

1. Esthetics and dermatology are services that ideally complement one another. The esthetician should be able to identify those skin disorders that may be treated in the salon and those that require medical attention.

   a) _Dermotologist_ is the study of the skin, its structure, its function, its diseases, and its treatment.

2. A lesion of the skin is a structural change in tissue caused by injury or damage. Name the characteristic primary lesion present in each of the following conditions.

   a) A discolored spot or patch that is neither raised or sunken is a _Macule_.

   b) A small, fluidless, elevated elevation of the skin is a _Papule_.

   c) An itchy, swollen lesion is called a _Wheal_.

   d) An abnormal solid lump larger than a papule is called a _Tubercle_.

   e) An external swelling from excessive cell multiplication that varies in shape and color is called a _Tumor_.

   f) A _Vesicles_ is a blister with clear fluid in it.

   g) A large blister containing a watery fluid similar to a vesicle is a _Bulla_.

   h) An elevation of the skin that is inflamed and contains pus is a _Pustule_.

3. Name the characteristic secondary lesions that develop in the later stages of a disease.

   a) A _Scale_ is an accumulation of epidermal flakes, dry or oily.

   b) A _Crust_ is an accumulation of sebum and pus mixed with other epidermal waste.

   c) A skin sore or abrasion caused by scratching or scraping the skin is called an _Excoriation_.

   d) A _Fissure_ is a crack in the skin that penetrates the dermis.

   e) An _ulcer_ is an open lesion on the skin or mucous membrane of the body, accompanied by pus and loss of skin depth.

   f) A _Scar_ is likely to form after the healing of a skin injury or condition.

WORD REVIEW

bulla	fissure	stain
contagious	lesion	subjective
crust	macule	tubercle
cyst	papule	tumor
dermatitis	pediculosis	venereal
dermatologist	pustule	vesicle
dermatology	scale	ulcer
epidemic	scar	wheal
excoriation		

RAPID REVIEW TEST

Date _____

Rating _____

Insert the correct term in the space provided.

abrasion	scale	ulcer
crust	secondary	vascular
dermatology	tertiary	wheal
keloid	tumors	

1. A scab is another name for a _____ crust _____ .

2. The subject of _____ dermatology _____ deals with diseases of the skin.

3. A thick scar resulting from excessive growth of tissue is a _____ Keloid _____ .

4. An epidermal flake is the same as a _____ scale _____ .

5. An open lesion of the skin or mucus membrane with loss of skin depth is an _____ ulcer _____ .

6. An insect bite causes a lesion known as a _____ wheal _____ .

7. Nodules are referred to as _____ Tumor _____ .

8. The esthetician is concerned with primary, ____ Secondary ____ , and ____ tertiary ____ skin lesions.

9. Another name for excoriation is _____ abrasion _____ .

10. Telangiectasia is an example of a _____ Vascular _____ lesion.

TOPIC 2: SEBACEOUS (OIL) GLAND DISORDERS

1. The common disorders of the sebaceous (oil) glands include whiteheads, blackheads, seborrhea, and acne. What is the medical term for each of the following skin conditions?

   a) Blackheads— *Comedone*

   b) Dry skin— *Asteatosis*

   c) Whiteheads— *Milia*

   d) Oily skin— *Sebaceous hyperplasias*

2. In cases of seborrhea, the sebaceous glands produce an excessive amount of oil.

   a) What is the appearance of the skin in this condition? *Severe oiliness of the skin*

   b) Describe sebaceous hyperplasias. *appear similar to open Comedones, are often donut shaped, with sebaceous material in the center. Cannot be removed by extraction, only Surgically.*

3. Acne is an inflammatory disorder of the skin involving the sebaceous glands. Is acne considered to be an acute or a chronic disease? *Yes.*

4. Rosacea is associated with redness and dilation of blood vessels of the skin.

   a) Where does rosacea usually appear on the face? *Cheeks and nose*

   b) What are three characteristics of rosacea?

      1. *Redness*

      2. *dilation of Blood vessels.*

      3. *The formation of papules and pustules*

5. A steatoma (also called a "wen" or "sebaceous cyst") is a subcutaneous tumor of the sebaceous glands.

   a) Where does steatoma usually occur? *It usually appears on the Scalp, neck and Back.*

   b) What are the characteristics of steatoma? *a sebaceous cyst filled with sebum which ranges in size from a pea to an orange.*

6. Asteatosis is a condition of dry, scaly skin. What is generally thought to be the cause of asteatosis? *Can be due to aging, body disorders, alkalies of harsh soaps, or Cold exposure*

7. A furuncle is caused by bacteria that enter the skin through the hair follicles.

    a) What is the commonly used term for furuncle? _____ *boils* _____

    b) What are the characteristics of a furuncle? _*a subcutaneous abscess filled with pus.*_

8. Give the primary indication of a cyst: _*a closed, abnormally developed sac containing fluid, infection*_

WORD REVIEW

acne	cyst	raised
acute	furuncle	rosacea
asteatosis debris	hair follicle	secretion
blackheads	lesion	sebaceous
clogged	milia	steatoma
chronic	pus	wen
comedones	pustule	whitehead

RAPID REVIEW TEST

Date: _____

Rating: _____

Place the correct word in spaces provided in the sentences below.

acne	milia	sebaceous hyperplasias
alkalies	rosacea	seborrhea
asteatosis	sebaceous	subcutaneous
comedones		

1. Blackheads are known as _____ *Comedones* _____.

2. Severe oiliness of the skin is referred to as _____ *Seborrhea* _____.

3. Asteatosis is a dry skin condition often caused by products containing _____ *alkalies* _____.

4. A furuncle is a _____ *Subcutaneous* _____ abscess filled with pus.

5. _____ *Sebaceous hyperplasias* _____ is an overgrowth of the sebaceous gland that can be only surgically removed.

6. Whiteheads are also known as _____ *milia* _____.

7. A chronic inflammatory disorder usually affecting the nose and cheeks is called _____ *Rosacea* _____.

8. A steatoma is also called a _____Sebaceous_____ cyst.

9. _____acne_____ is a chronic inflammatory disorder of the sebaceous glands.

10. A dry skin due to aging or body disorder is known as _____asteatosis_____.

TOPIC 3: DISORDERS AND IMPERFECTIONS OF THE SKIN

1. Although the esthetician cannot diagnose nor treat disorders of the sudoriferous (sweat) glands, it is important to understand that these disorders can produce abnormal changes in the sweat production of the body. Which disorders are associated with the following?

    a) Miliaria rubra _____

    b) Bromhidrosis _____

    c) Hyperhidrosis _____

    d) Lack of perspiration _____

2. *Dermatitis* refers to an inflammatory condition of the skin. List three types of skin lesions that are usually found in dermatitis.

    a) _____

    b) _____

    c) _____

3. Eczema is a form of dermatitis that should be treated by a physician. What are the two basic signs of eczema?

    a) _____

    b) _____

4. Psoriasis is a common chronic inflammatory disease. What are the usual signs of psoriasis?

    _____

5. Herpes simplex is a viral infection commonly identified as fever blisters. Where do the blisters usually appear? _____Blisters usually appear on the lips or nostrils_____

6. Abnormal conditions involving skin pigmentation may result from internal or external causes. Match the proper term with the following definition.

albinism   lentigines   nevus
chloasma   leucoderma   tan
hyperpigmentation

a) _tan_   Exposure to the sun.

b) _lentigines_   Small spots called freckles (usually red or yellow-brown).

c) _chloasma_   Increased pigmentation commonly called "liver spots".

d) _nevus_   Dark stain commonly called a "birthmark".

e) _Leucoderma_   Abnormal light patches on the skin.

f) _albinism_   Congenital condition of the skin when it lacks color pigment.

g) _hyperpigmentation_ Overproduction of pigment.

7. Hypertrophies are excessive or new growths on the skin. Match the proper term with the following definition.

actinic keratoses   keratosis pilaris   skin tag
keratoma   mole   verruca

a) _Keratoma_   Acquired thickened patch of epidermis.

b) _mole_   Brownish spot that can be flat or raised.

c) _Verruca_   Commonly called a "wart."

d) _Skin tag_   Small flap-like extension of the skin.

e) _actinic Keratoses_ Rough, pink or flesh-toned precancerous lesions from sun damage.

f) _Keratosis pilaris_ Bumpiness in cheeks and upperarms.

WORD REVIEW

albinism	hyperhidrosis	pigment
anhidrosis	lentigines	psoriasis
birthmark	leucoderma	skin tags
bromhidrosis	miliaria rubra	stain
chloasma	mole	sudoriferous
dermatitis	nevus	venenata
eczema	papules	verruca
herpes simplex	perspiration	vitiligo

RAPID REVIEW TEST

Date: _____

Rating: _____

Insert the correct term in the space provided. Some terms may be used more than once.

albinism ✓

anhidrosis ✓

bromhidrosis ✓

chloasma ✓

contact dermatitis ✓

dermatitis

edema ✓

erythema ✓

herpes simplex ✓

hyperhidrosis

keratoma ✓

leucoderma ✓

lentigines ✓

melasma ✓

miliaria rubra ✓

nevus ✓

psoriasis ✓

sudoriferous ✓

venenata ✓

1. When excessive sweating occurs, it is called ___bromhidrosis___.

2. ___Chloasma___ is a condition commonly referred to as "liver spots."

3. The absence of melanin pigment in the body is called ___albinism___.

4. ___Psoriasis___ is a skin condition characterized by silvery scales.

5. Allergic reactions from contact with a substance or chemicals is called ___Contact dermatitis___.

6. Swelling is called ___edema___.

7. A birthmark is also referred to as a ___Nevus___.

8. A burning or itching sensation of the skin which may be caused by excessive heat is a sign of _____ ___Miliaria ruba___.

9. When the body lacks perspiration, it is called ___Anhidrosis___.

10. The "mask of pregnancy" is often referred to as ___Melasma___.

11. When perspiration has a strong, disagreeable order, the condition is called _____.

12. Redness caused by inflammation is called ___erythema___.

13. Prickly heat is also called _____.

14. _____Dermatitis._____ is the medical term for various forms of lesions affecting the skin.

15. Occupational disorders such as dermatitis _____Venenata_____ may be caused by chemicals.

16. _____Lentigenes._____ is the medical term for freckles.

17. An acquired overgrowth of epidermis is a _____Keratoma_____ of the skin.

18. _____Leucoderma_____ refers to light patches or colorless areas of the skin.

19. The _____Sudoriferous_____ glands are commonly called sweat glands.

20. Fever blisters are often the sign of _____Herpes Simplex_____.

TOPIC 4: OTHER SERIOUS DISORDERS OF THE SKIN

1. The esthetician helps the client keep his or her skin clean and healthy. When a skin condition is obviously in need of medical treatment, it may be necessary to suggest to the client that he or she consult a physician.

   a) The least malignant and most common cancer is called basal cell _____Carcinoma_____, often characterized by _____light_____, _____pearly_____ nodules.

   b) The most serious skin cancer is called malignant _____Melanoma_____.

   c) _____Squamous._____ cell carcinoma is characterized by scaly red papules or nodules.

2. Insert the proper term in the space provided for the following definitions with the illustration that it correctly describes.

abrasion	laceration	scar
cyst	nodule /	ulcer /
fissure	polyp	
incision	puncture	

An _____ is rough and red where the skin has been scraped or worn away.

A _____ is a growth that extends from the surface of the skin. They may also grow within the body.

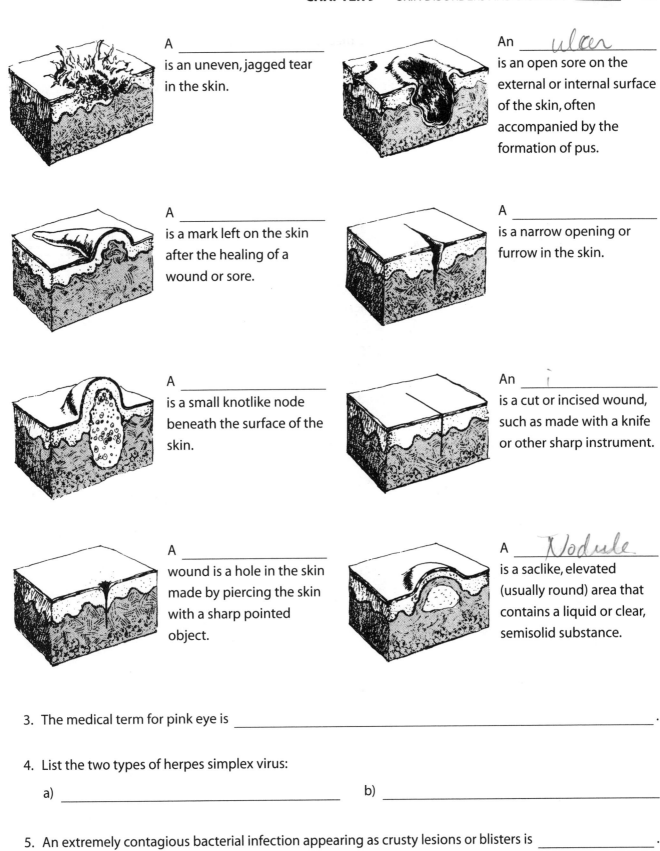

A _____ is an uneven, jagged tear in the skin.

An ___ulcer___ is an open sore on the external or internal surface of the skin, often accompanied by the formation of pus.

A _____ is a mark left on the skin after the healing of a wound or sore.

A _____ is a narrow opening or furrow in the skin.

A _____ is a small knotlike node beneath the surface of the skin.

An ___i___ is a cut or incised wound, such as made with a knife or other sharp instrument.

A _____ wound is a hole in the skin made by piercing the skin with a sharp pointed object.

A ___Nodule___ is a saclike, elevated (usually round) area that contains a liquid or clear, semisolid substance.

3. The medical term for pink eye is _____.

4. List the two types of herpes simplex virus:

   a) _____   b) _____

5. An extremely contagious bacterial infection appearing as crusty lesions or blisters is _____.

6. The professional term for fungal infections is _____.

7. Name the two terms for a yeast infection that prevents melanin production.

   a) _____   b) _____

8. Verruca refers to _____.

WORD REVIEW

abrasion	eczema	regenerate
allergy	epidermis	scar
basal cell carcinoma	fissure	sensitivity
benign	hives	syphilis
cancer	incision laceration	tumor
cyst	malignant melanoma	ulcer
degeneration	nodule	venenata
dermatitis	polyp	
drugs	puncture	

10

SKIN ANALYSIS

Date: _____

Rating: _____

Text Pages: 206–223

TOPIC 1: CONSULTATION AND SKIN ANALYSIS

Before performing services or selecting products, skin types and conditions must be analyzed correctly.

1. List two benefits of a thorough analysis.

   a) _____

   b) _____

2. _____ and _____ factors contribute to the skin's condition.

3. In addition to physically looking and feeling the skin, list three additional items necessary for comprehensive analysis.

   a) _____   c) _____

   b) _____

TOPIC 2: SKIN TYPES

1. _____ and _____ generally determine the type of skin.

2. Skin that is lacking oil is considered as being _____.

3. Generally, what size are the pores of dry skin? _____

4. What is the purpose of occlusive products? _____

5. Describe the difference between "dry skin" and "dehydrated skin." _____

   _____

6. Describe the characteristics of the pores of normal skin. _____

   _____

7. Of what purpose would a skin care regimen have for a normal skin type? _____

   _____

8. Combination skin can be both _____ and _____ at the same time.

9. List the three areas that are included in the T-zone.

   a) _____   c) _____

   b) _____

10. What type of products is best suited for combination skin? _____

11. List two characteristics of oily skin.

    a) _____

    b) _____

12. What is the goal when treating this type of skin? _____

13. What can make oily skin worse? _____

    Why? _____

    _____

14. Sensitive skin is both a _____ and _____ .

15. What three factors can aggravate sensitive skin?

    a) _____

    b) _____

    c) _____

16. Sensitive skin is characterized by _____ , and is easily irritated.

17. Put the letter that corresponds with the correct answer in the space provided.

    _____ Tans   a) Very fair; light-colored eyes and hair, freckles common

    _____ Always burns, never tans   b) Mideastern skin; rarely sun sensitive

    _____ Sometimes burns, gradual   c) Black skin, rarely sun sensitive
              tanning

    _____ Burns easily   d) Mediterrranean Caucasian; medium to heavy pigmentation

    _____ Tans easily   e) Fair skinned; light eyes; light hair

    _____ Rarely burns, always tans   f) Very common skin type; fair; eye and hair varies

18. Black skin needs more exfoliation and deep pore cleansing due to its susceptibility to _____
_____ .

19. What ethnic skin is considered as one of the most sensitive? _____

RAPID REVIEW TEST

Date: _____

Rating: _____

Insert the correct term in the space provided.

alipidic	fragile	melanin
color	hyperpigmentation	sensitive
dehydrated		

1. Skin lacking oil is called _____ .

2. Skin that is _____ can be found in all skin types.

3. Low tolerance to products and stimulation are characteristics of _____ skin.

4. _____ gives the skin its _____ and protection from the sun.

5. Darker skin is prone to _____ .

6. Insert the correct term in the space provided.

acneic	dry	normal
combination	mature/aging	oily
couperose		

a) _____ skin in good condition with a sufficient supply of sebum and moisture

b) _____ skin having both dry and oily areas

c) _____ skin lacking oil or moisture or both

d) _____ skin generally loose, wrinkled, or lined

e) _____ skin identified by broken capillaries

f) _____ skin with an overabundance of sebum

g) _____ blemished skin

TOPIC 3: SKIN CONDITIONS

Many internal and external factors affect the condition of the skin.

1. What are the most common conditions of the skin that an esthetician focuses on? Name six.

    a) _____

    b) _____

    c) _____

    d) _____

    e) _____

    f) _____

2. Explain the difference between open and closed comedones. _____

    _____

3. Milia is the professional term for _____ , and must be removed by _____ .

4. Habits, diet, and stress affect the health and appearance of our body and skin. List four major causes of skin conditions.

    a) _____   c) _____

    b) _____   d) _____

5. There are many internal and external factors that cause skin conditions. Place an "I" for intrinsic or "E" for extrinsic in the space provided for each of the following causes below.

    _____ 1. dehydration   _____ 8. misuse of products or treatments

    _____ 2. smoking/alcohol   _____ 9. sun damage

    _____ 3. genetics/ethnicity   _____ 10. metal pins

    _____ 4. poor maintenance/home care   _____ 11. ingredient intolerance/allergies

    _____ 5. environment/humidity   _____ 12. pregnancy, heart conditions

    _____ 6. stress   _____ 13. lack of rest/exercise

    _____ 7. pollutants   _____ 14. free radicals

6. If it is illegal to ask clients about contagious diseases, how can you find out if there is a potential contraindication? _____

    _____

7. Give four things you will look for during a skin analysis.

a) _____   c) _____

b) _____   d) _____

8. Why is it important to look at the client's skin type and conditions prior to cleansing?

_____

WORD REVIEW

abnormalities	cysts	magnifying lamp
allergy	diagnose	medication
analyze	examine	microcirculation
asphyxiated	eyepads	occlusive
atmosphere	flakiness	sanitize
comedone	follicle	texture
condition	hydrated	T-zone
contraindication	keratosis	Wood's lamp
consultation	lipids	

RAPID REVIEW TEST

Date: _____

Rating: _____

Insert the correct term in the space provided.

asphyxiated	contraindications	sanitized
clogged	hyperkeratinization	several
consultation	hyperpigmentation	sun
contagious	hypopigmentation	Wood's

1. _____ and _____ are two pigmentation disorders common to the esthetician.

2. An excessive build-up of dead skin cells is referred to as _____.

3. _____ skin is due to lack of oxygen, characterized by _____ pores.

4. The _____ is the cause of approximately 80 percent of aging.

5. Medications, contagious diseases, skin disorders, and irritation are _____ of a service.

6. Services on a client are prohibited if the client has a _____ disease.

7. It is important to include a client _____ during the analysis.

8. A noticeable improvement of the condition may take _____ treatments.

9. The _____ lamp is used to detect dehydration, sun damage, and other disorders of the skin.

10. The esthetician's hands should be _____ before the skin is analyzed.

ACTIVITY

Choose a skin type such as dry, oily, combination, mature, or a specific condition, and design a brochure that you could give to your client. In this brochure, describe the condition and give the proper care and maintenance of the type. Include any precautions, contraindications, and so forth. You may want to make an area for a schedule of appointments and treatment therapies that you determine necessary for the chosen skin type. Make the brochure appealing to the eye, so clients will want to read and follow the instructions listed.

11

PRODUCT SELECTION AND INGREDIENTS

Date: _____

Rating: _____

Text pages: 224–257

TOPIC 1: PRODUCTS

1. Name the five main categories in skin care products.

   a) _____

   b) _____

   c) _____

   d) _____

   e) _____

2. Why is soap not usually recommended as a cleanser? _____

   _____

3. What are the three basic forms of cleansers?

   a) _____

   b) _____

   c) _____

4. Give two reasons why you should practice caution when prescribing a foaming wash.

   a) _____

   b) _____

5. List three benefits of cleansers.

   a) _____

   b) _____

   c) _____

6. Tonic lotions include _____ , _____ , and _____ .

7. Why do you include tonic lotions to your facial procedure? List four reasons.

a) _____

b) _____

c) _____

d) _____

8. An exfoliant is an ingredient that assists in what process? _____

_____

9. What are the two basic types of exfoliation treatments?

a) _____

b) _____

10. Granular scrubs and brushing machines are examples of which type of exfoliation treatment? _____

_____

11. List five types of skin that should not be mechanically exfoliated.

a) _____

b) _____

c) _____

d) _____

e) _____

12. Alphahydroxy acids and enzymes are samples of what type of exfoliation treatment? _____

13. Gommage is removed from the skin by _____.

14. Why are peels beneficial to the skin?

a) _____

b) _____

15. Over-exfoliating will cause _____ .

16. Masks and packs offer many benefits. List seven advantages of using these products.

    a) _____

    b) _____

    c) _____

    d) _____

    e) _____

    f) _____

    g) _____

17. What is added to masks to create healing and antiseptic properties? _____

18. Masks and packs are generally allowed to stay on the skin for approximately _____ minutes.

19. Paraffin wax masks are used to _____ and
    _____ .

20. What is another name for thermal masks? _____

21. What causes the increased temperature in thermal masks? _____
    _____

22. When do you apply serums? _____

23. Why do serums penetrate deeper into the skin? _____

24. Lotions, hydrators, and creams are known as _____ .

25. Why does oily skin need hydration? _____
    _____

26. What is the function of humectants? _____

27. Sun exposure is damaging to the skin. What six negative results can occur when the skin is not protected from ultraviolet rays?

a) _____

b) _____

c) _____

d) _____

e) _____

f) _____

28. Sunscreen with an SPF of 8 blocks _____ percent of the UVB rays, while an SPF of 30 blocks _____ percent.

29. What is the active ingredient in self-tanning lotion? _____

VOCABULARY REVIEW

Date: _____

Rating: _____

antioxidants	jojoba	retinoic acid
binders	licorice	silicone
emollients	mineral oil	solvents
glycerin	petroleum jelly	witch hazel

1. _____ lie on the surface to prevent water loss.

2. A nonallergenic emollient, cleanser, and demulsifier is _____ .

3. _____ are topically applied and neutralized free radicals.

4. _____ is an anti-irritant and used for sensitive skin.

5. _____ is used after laser surgery to protect the skin while healing.

6. _____ are substances that hold products together.

7. _____ dissolve other ingredients.

8. _____ is a skin softener, humectant, and a water binder.

9. _____ is an oil extracted from the bean-like seeds of a desert shrub.

10. _____ is an emollient that leaves a protective film on the surface of the skin.

11. _____ is extracted from the bark of the hamanelis shrub.

12. _____ is derived from vitamin A and has the ability to alter collagen.

RAPID REVIEW TEST

Date: _____

Rating: _____

Insert the correct term in the space provided.

antimicrobial	exfoliating	pH
concentrated	hypoallergenic	titanium dioxide
consultation	oily	ultraviolet
emulsions		

1. An _____ agent is sometimes added to face washes to kill bacteria.

2. Fresheners and toners can restore the _____ balance of the skin.

3. When _____ , care must be taken not to damage the capillaries.

4. Moisturizers are _____ that protect the barrier layer.

5. Emollients are not usually recommended for _____ skin types.

6. Ampules contain _____ active ingredients.

7. An example of a physical sun-block is _____ .

8. When prescribing a home regimen, it is important to do a client _____ .

9. _____ ingredients are used to reduce allergic reactions.

10. _____ rays are damaging to the skin and can cause cancer.

ACTIVITY

Using the charts in your textbook, develop a home regimen plan for oily, normal, dry, mature, sensitive, acneic, and combination skin types. Get creative! (These products do not have to exist, you may create them.) Use herbs, oils, extracts, and so on as additives (example: toner with spearmint extract).

12

THE TREATMENT ROOM

Date: _____

Rating: _____

Text pages: 252–268

INTRODUCTION

1. To provide quality service, the esthetician must be _____ and _____ .

2. List six characteristics both mental and physical that a professional should portray to be successful.

   a) _____

   b) _____

   c) _____

   d) _____

   e) _____

   f) _____

TOPIC 1: FURNITURE AND EQUIPMENT

1. A basic treatment room should consist of the following basic equipment:

   a) _____

   b) _____

   c) _____

   d) _____

   e) _____

   f) _____

   g) _____

   h) _____

   i) _____

   j) _____

2. A separate room for mixing products and storing supplies is called a _____ .

3. The treatment room should be equipped with at least a basic complement of supplies. List twelve items that should be available to the esthetician.

a) _____   h) _____

b) _____   i) _____

c) _____   j) _____

d) _____   k) _____

e) _____   l) _____

f) _____   m) _____

g) _____

4. Briefly describe the process for making cleansing pads. _____
_____
_____

5. What are the two types of eye pads?

a) _____

b) _____

6. How do you determine the correct size of eye pad? _____
_____

7. Summarize the making of eye pads . _____
_____

8. List eight of the basic products used in the facial procedures.

a) _____   e) _____

b) _____   f) _____

c) _____   g) _____

d) _____   h) _____

9. Describe the basic steps to prepare the facial bed for a client.

a) _____

b) _____

c) _____

d) _____

e) _____

10. The study of adapting work conditions to suit the worker is called _____.

11. Where should clean items be stored? _____

12. How should you prepare the work surface to receive supplies? _____
_____

WORD REVIEW

biohazard	ergonomic	sanitary
bolster	extraction	sharps container
disposable	OSHA	

RAPID REVIEW TEST

Date: _____

Rating: _____

Insert the correct term in the space provided.

airtight	client safety	esthetically
biohazard or Sharps	closed	state sanitation regulations
butterfly	comfortable	used
clean	distilled	vinyl

1. A treatment room should be _____ pleasing.

2. The most important considerations before, during, and after treatment are _____
and _____.

3. To prevent back and hand problems, make sure the work area is _____.

4. _____ gloves are recommended for use with products containing oils.

5. Unused prepared pads can be stored in an _____ container.

6. _____ pads will not fall from eyes as easily.

7. What type of water is used for the steamer? _____

8. Never store wet brushes in a _____ container.

9. Place soiled disposable items in a _____ container.

10. Do not mix _____ and _____ items.

13

MASSAGE

Date: _____

Rating: _____

Text pages: 270–285

TOPIC 1: THE BENEFITS OF MASSAGE

1. a) Massage is one of the oldest therapeutic methods. Be aware of the state regulations regarding massage as an esthetician. Massage has both _____ and _____ benefits.

   b) What four areas of the body is an esthetician's massage limited to?

   1. _____   3. _____

   2. _____   4. _____

2. Facial massage has many benefits. List ten positive results from facial massage.

   a) _____   f) _____

   b) _____   g) _____

   c) _____   h) _____

   d) _____   i) _____

   e) _____   j) _____

3. Hand movements should be _____ and glide _____ from one area to the next.

4. Hand _____ is one way to prevent carpal tunnel syndrome for the technician.

5. What are five conditions of the body or skin that would contraindicate massage?

   a) _____   d) _____

   b) _____   e) _____

   c) _____

6. What care should be taken with the arthritic client? _____

7. List five massage movements used in massage.

a) _____   d) _____

b) _____   e) _____

c) _____

8. The most important and widely used movement is _____ .

9. Chucking, rolling, and wringing are variations of which movement? _____

10. Generally, massage movements are directed from _____ toward the _____ of the muscle.

11. One way to learn which techniques feel good and which do not is to _____ .

12. If it is necessary to remove your hands from the client's face during a massage, you should _____ _____ .

TOPIC 2: TYPES OF MASSAGE MOVEMENTS

1. Write the definition of the word in the space provided.

a) Effleurage _____
_____

b) Petrissage _____

c) Friction _____
_____

d) Tapotement _____

e) Vibration _____

2. a) Three variations of friction movements are _____ , _____ , and _____ .

b) Where do you use these types of friction movements? _____

3. _____ effleurage is used on smaller surfaces such as the _____ or _____ .

4. _____ effleurage is used on larger areas such as the _____ or _____ .

5. Friction movement _____ circulation and glandular activity.

6. What movement usually begins and ends a massage sequence? _____

7. _____ is the most stimulating of the general movements, and should be used _____.

_____.

8. Describe how slapping movements are performed. _____

_____

9. a) What part of the hands do you use when executing hacking movements? _____

_____

   b) The parts of the body that you use in hacking and slapping movements are the _____,

   _____ , and _____.

10. Vibration is a highly stimulating movement, and should never be used more than a _____ in one spot.

RAPID REVIEW TEST

Date: _____

Rating: _____

Complete these sentences with the words listed below.

acupressure	friction	reflexology
aromatherapy	Jacquet	rolling
chucking	lymph drainage massage	vibration
effleurage	petrissage	wringing

1. _____ encourages the removal of waste from the body.

2. A kneading movement that stimulates the underlying tissues is _____.

3. As the hands are working downward, the flesh is twisted against the bones in opposite directions during

_____.

4. A technique named after a French dermatologist is _____.

5. A method of applying pressure to points on the body to release muscle tension is _____.

6. Both hands moving at the same time opposite to each other twisting the flesh up and down the bone is referred to as _____.

7. Pressure is maintained on the skin while the fingers or palms are moved over the underlying structures defines _____.

8. _____ is the soft continuous stroking movement applied with the fingers and palms.

9. When the flesh is grasped in one hand and moved up and down along the bone while the other hand steadies the arm is called _____.

10. _____ is a technique that is accomplished by rapid muscular contractions in the arms.

11. _____ is a technique that uses essential oils that penetrate the skin during massage movements.

12. _____ is similar to acupressure; manipulates areas on the hands and feet.

14

BASIC FACIALS AND TREATMENTS

Date: _____

Rating: _____

Text pages: 286–321

TOPIC 1: FACIAL TREATMENT BENEFITS

1. What are the general benefits of skin treatments?

   a) _____

   b) _____

   c) _____

2. What must a professional have in order to be successful?

   a) _____

   b) _____

   c) _____

3. What are five contraindications of giving facial treatments?

   a) _____   d) _____

   b) _____   e) _____

   c) _____

4. Briefly summarize the draping process.

   a) _____

   b) _____

   c) _____

   d) _____

   e) _____

5. List the nine steps of the facial process.

a) _____   f) _____

b) _____   g) _____

c) _____   h) _____

d) _____   i) _____

e) _____

6. _____ cleansers are desirable during facials.

7. The product that should be used for lip color removal is _____ and it should be applied by _____ .

8. What three benefits are found in the exfoliation process?

a) _____

b) _____

c) _____

9. Heat applied through steam or warm towels accomplishes what five things?

a) _____

b) _____

c) _____

d) _____

e) _____

10. Once properly trained, the skin care professional will accomplish what two goals by performing extractions?

a) _____   b) _____

11. What implements are used to perform extractions?

a) _____   b) _____

12. What areas have follicular walls perpendicular to the surface of the skin?

    a) _____   c) _____

    b) _____   d) _____

13. What products can be used to help soften the plugs of cells?

    a) _____   b) _____

14. A small gage needle used to help the extraction process is called a _____ .

15. Most clients will tolerate approximately _____ minutes of extraction.

16. For the following areas, give the proper extraction procedure.

    a) Chin— _____

    b) Nose— _____

    _____

    c) Cheeks— _____

    d) Forehead, upper cheekbones— _____

17. Give the proper use of a lancet when opening closed comedones. _____

_____

18. List the four steps when preparing for manual extractions.

    a) _____

    b) _____

    c) _____

    d) _____

19. _____ should be worn at all times during the above procedures.

20. Describe the benefits of the treatment mask.

    a) _____   d) _____

    b) _____   e) _____

    c) _____   f) _____

21. List the steps to a basic facial.

a) _____   f) _____

b) _____   g) _____

c) _____   h) _____

d) _____   i) _____

e) _____   j) _____

22. _____ are concentrated ingredients used for specific corrective treatments.

23. The purposes of moisturizers are _____
_____ .

24. _____ are antioxidants that are recommended for aging or sun-dried skin.

25. The hydrating ingredients that are recommended for aging skin are _____
_____ .

26. The facial treatment used on sensitive skin should be _____ .

27. List several salon treatments that may be offered to clients to help improve acne skin.

a) _____   f) _____

b) _____   g) _____

c) _____   h) _____

d) _____   i) _____

e) _____

WORD REVIEW

antioxidants

benzyl peroxide

capillaries

contraindications

debris

exfoliation

extraction

facial zones

FDA

glycolic peel

hydrate

lancet

protocol

serums

skin histology

trauma

vasodilators

RAPID REVIEW TEST

Date: _____

Rating: _____

Insert the correct term in the space provided.

contraindications	laundry costs	sanitation
draping	rejuvenate	serums
extractions	remove	steps
facial sponges		

1. A facial is a professional service designed to improve and _____ .

2. _____ are conditions that would prevent the client from being able to receive a treatment.

3. _____ the client refers to adjusting the head drape, towels, and linens.

4. An esthetician should consider efficiency and _____ when determining what to use for draping.

5. Because foam or gel cleansers are harder to _____ , it is advisable to use a milky or creamy cleanser.

6. While cleansing, some estheticians prefer to use wet cotton pads, and others choose to use _____ _____ .

7. The skin must be exfoliated and warmed prior to _____ .

8. _____ are concentrated ingredients used for specific treatments.

9. Performing your _____ procedures in the presence of your client will cause them to feel more confident in you as a professional.

10. The main differences between a mini-facial and a basic facial are the time and the number of _____ .

TOPIC 2: MEN'S SKIN CARE

1. List the key points to consider when choosing skin care products for men.

    a) _____

    b) _____

2. What two applications should not be used on freshly shaved skin?

   a) _____

   b) _____

3. What type of protective clothing do men wear during a treatment? _____

_____

RAPID REVIEW

Date: _____

Rating: _____

Insert the correct term in the space provided.

basic facial	paraffin wax	treatment plan
continuous	privately	water-based
enzyme peel	razor bumps	
hyperpigmentation	shaving	

1. A skin treatment follows the same procedures as the _____ .

2. To treat dry skin, a thermal or _____ mask should be used.

3. An _____ formulated for sensitive skin is a gentle way to exfoliate sensitive skin.

4. Sun exposure causes dark pigmentation spots on the skin called _____ .

5. In order to make male clients feel more comfortable, the consultation should take place _____ .

6. _____ before a man's facial makes the skin more sensitive.

7. Pseudofolliculitis is also known as _____ .

8. Working with problem skin is a _____ process and clients need to follow regular skin care programs.

9. Oily and combination skins need _____ products.

10. The esthetician can outline a _____ to help bring acne skin into a normal functioning condition.

15

MACHINES

Date: _____

Rating: _____

Text pages: 322–343

INTRODUCTION

1. Electrical devices can enhance skin analysis, product penetration, and skin sanitation. The use of devices for therapeutic benefits is called _____ .

2. It is important to be aware of current technology to maintain _____ with your clients.

TOPIC 1: SKIN CARE EQUIPMENT

1. The magnifying lamp is used to assist in analysis of the skin and to treat the skin.

   a) The magnifying lamp is also known as a _____ .

   b) What type of light bulb is used in the lamp? _____

   c) The unit of measure used to indicate the strength of magnification is known as _____ .

   d) _____ can be used to protect the client's eyes from the bright light.

   e) The lens of the magnifying lamp should be cleaned by spraying with a disinfectant and wiping with a

   _____ .

2. a) The Wood's lamp is a _____ light used to eliminate skin _____ .

   b) _____ , _____ , and _____
   are three kinds of disorders a Wood's lamp can help identify.

   c) The Wood's lamp must be used in a totally _____ room.

3. a) The rotary brush is used to lightly _____ and _____ the skin.

   b) The brush machine should be used in a circular pattern beginning on the _____ and
   ending in the _____ area.

   c) Brushes should be immersed into a _____ and stored
   in a _____ after drying.

4. a) What are the two main functions of the vacuum (suction) machine?

    1. _____

    2. _____

  b) The vacuum helps to stimulate the skin by _____ .

  c) Vacuuming should not be used on _____ ,

    _____ , _____ , or _____ skin.

  d) The vacuum spray is used to _____ and _____ the skin.

  e) The sprayer can be filled with _____ or _____ to mist the client's face.

5. a) What are five benefits of using a steamer?

    1. _____   3. _____

    2. _____   4. _____

  b) Ordinary treatment time for the steamer is between _____ and _____ minutes.

  c) Too much steam can cause skin to become _____ .

  d) _____ are highly active and should never be placed in the steamer water.

  e) If not properly maintained, a steamer can become clogged and, as a result, _____ .

  f) What substance is best for cleaning the steamer? _____

6. a. The Lucas sprayer is designed to apply the following:

    1. _____   4. _____

    2. _____   5. _____

    3. _____

  b) The Lucas sprayer emits a mist that is _____ and _____ and is beneficial to

    _____ , _____ , and _____ skin types.

WORD REVIEW

aromatherapy	distortion	therapeutic
diopter	exfoliate	velocity contraindication
disincrustation	oxygenate	
distilled	ozone	

RAPID REVIEW TEST

Date: _____

Rating: _____

Insert the correct term in the space provided.

cool	essential oils	shape
dehydrated	fifteen	spit
distilled	oiliness	white
distortion	ozone	yellow
dryness		

1. Without a clear lens, _____ will add strain to your eyes when using the mag light.

2. A Wood's lamp allows the esthetician to see the _____
   and _____ of the skin.

3. Rotary brushes must be dried in a way that they do not lose their _____ .

4. Steamers with _____ have an antiseptic effect on the skin.

5. When steam is used, it should be kept _____ inches from the skin.

6. _____ may cause the steamer's glass to break from pressure if used in the water.

7. Mineral deposits cause a steamer to _____ hot water, and may cause burns.

8. _____ water is recommended for use in the steamer.

9. Mineral deposit build-up appears as a _____ or _____ crusty film.

10. Lucas sprayers emit a _____ mist, which is beneficial to _____ skin.

TOPIC 2: ELECTRICAL TOOLS AND OTHER EQUIPMENT

1. a) The high-frequency machine produces between _____ and _____ Hertz frequency.

   b) Because it changes polarity 1,000 times per second, it has _____ and _____ produce a chemical change.

   c) The high-frequency machine provides what six benefits?

   1. _____   4. _____

   2. _____   5. _____

   3. _____   6. _____

2. a) What two reactions are expected with the use of galvanic current?

   1. _____

   2. _____

   b) Disincrustation is used for _____ cleansing.

   c) During disincrustation, the sebum of the skin is transformed into soap in a process known as

   _____ .

   d) Iontophoresis allows the esthetician to introduce _____ products into the skin using electricity.

3. a) The heat mask delivers deep penetrating _____ heat through the layers of the skin.

   b) It is used in place of _____ or _____ for deep cleaning and softening of the skin.

4. a) Another term for microcurrent is _____ .

   b) It is used to treat what two conditions?

   1. _____   2. _____

   c) What reaction is visible when a microcurrent treatment is performed? _____

   _____

   d) Microcurrrent is intended to accomplish what four benefits?

   1. _____   3. _____

   2. _____   4. _____

5. a) Microdermabrasion is a powerful _____ .

    b) Briefly, explain the process of microdermabrasion. _____

       _____

    c) Microcrystals are composed of _____ .

    d) List six benefits of using microdermabrasion for exfoliation.

       1. _____   4. _____

       2. _____   5. _____

       3. _____   6. _____

6. _____ and _____ are absolutely mandatory for the use of microdermabrasion.

7. Laser skin resurfacing can be directed to _____ the surface of the skin without touching the lower _____ .

8. What two types of light rays are used for light therapy?

    a) _____

    b) _____

RAPID REVIEW TEST

Date: _____

Rating: _____

Insert the correct term in the space provided.

anaphoresis	galvanic	saponification
cataphoresis	microdermabrasion	sinusoidal
electrical	positive	thermolysis
electrode		

1. _____ current is used with high frequency.

2. _____ uses a stronger high frequency for permanent hair removal.

3. By converting oscillating current from an outlet to direct current, the _____ current creates a relaxation response to nerve endings.

4. When performing disincrustation, the client holds the _____ electrode, and the esthetician has direct contact with the disincrustor that is set on positive polarity.

5. The _____ must be directly on the skin before turning on the galvanic machine.

6. Ions carry an _____ charge.

7. _____ is the penetration of a positive product.

8. _____ is the infusion of a negative product.

9. An infra-ray mask will cause _____ .

10. _____ is a new form of exfoliation, and requires additional training.

16

HAIR REMOVAL

Date: _____

Rating: _____

Text pages: 344–379

TOPIC 1: ELECTROLYSIS AND OTHER METHODS OF REMOVING UNWANTED HAIR

1. The removal of superfluous hair is a service offered by most salons.

   a) What is the difference between temporary and permanent methods of hair removal? _____

   _____

   _____

   b) Two methods most frequently used for permanent hair reduction are _____
   and _____.

   c) What are five popular methods for temporary removal of superfluous hair?

      1. _____

      2. _____

      3. _____

      4. _____

      5. _____

   d) The temporary method commonly used to shape eyebrows is _____.

   e) The three stages of hair growth are _____, _____,
   and _____.

2. Match the definitions with the terminology from the list below.

   barbae folliculitis   hirsutism   temporary hair removal
   electrologist   hypertrichosis   trichology
   epilation   laser hair removal

   a) _____ removes hair for a short period of time.

   b) _____ is a person trained, licensed, or certified to perform permanent
   hair reduction.

   c) _____ is the removal of hair by the roots.

   d) _____ is the same as ingrown hairs.

e) _____ is increased growth of hair in areas where it is not normal.

f) _____ uses light/heat influences in the destruction of the hair papilla.

g) _____ is a condition influenced by an imbalance of hormones in which density and amount of hair increases beyond normal.

h) _____ is the scientific study of hair and its diseases.

3. It is important for the esthetician to understand the structure of the hair.

   a) What is the purpose of hair? _____

   b) Where do the cells necessary for hair growth originate? _____

   c) The main structures of the hair root below the surface are _____ , _____ , _____ , and _____ .

   d) Disulfide bonds are broken by _____ .

   e) Where are supercilia hairs found? _____

   f) The soft, fine hair covering the body is referred to as _____ or _____ .

4. Curly, wavy, and straight hair are determined by the angle of the hair follicle. Why is it important for electrologists to analyze the hair characteristics? _____ _____

5. a) _____ is the stage when the hair bulb is not active, resting.

   b) During the _____ stage, hair grows at a normal rate, with activity in the hair bulb.

6. A person who wants to practice electrolysis must be thoroughly trained in the most up-to-date methods. The areas of the face and body that should never receive electrolysis are _____ , _____ , _____ , and _____ .

   When tweezing, *firmly* pull the hair at a _____ .

7. Wax hair removal treatments are popular salon services.

   a) The two types of waxes are _____ and _____ .

   b) What do both waxes have in common? _____

8. a) A _____ is required prior to waxing service.

   b) What conditions of the skin would prohibit waxing? List eight.

   1. _____   5. _____

   2. _____   6. _____

   3. _____   7. _____

   4. _____   8. _____

   c) When the wax method is used to remove hair from the upper lip, in which direction is the fiber strip pulled? _____

9. Wax should not be used when clients are on certain medications. Name five medications that may cause concern.

   a) _____   d) _____

   b) _____   e) _____

   c) _____

10. a) Damage to the hair follicle during a hair removal procedure can result in _____ and _____ .

    b) What is the purpose of wearing gloves during services? _____
    _____

    c) Why is "double dipping" into the wax prohibited? _____
    _____

11. If hair is too long, what should you do before applying the wax? _____

12. List the three most important procedures during the wax removal.

    a) _____

    b) _____

    c) _____

13. a) What direction is the wax applied? _____

    b) What direction is the wax removed (both hard and soft)? _____
    _____

WORD REVIEW

adhere	hair growth rate	regrowth
bonding	hair texture	shaving
diabetic	heredity	skin test
diathermy	high-frequency	soft wax
dormant hair	hirsuties	stubble
electrologist	hirsutism	superfluous
electrolysis	hormone	talcum powder
epilation	hypertrichosis	tea tree
fabric strip	lanugo (fine) hair tweezing	temporary
galvanic	muslin	thermolysis
growth angle	papilla	wax method
hair growth direction	permanent hair removal	wax pot

RAPID REVIEW TEST

Date: _____

Rating: _____

Insert the proper term in the space provided.

depilatories	hirsutism	temporary
electrolysis	hypertrichosis	thermolysis
epilation	permanent	
galvanic	superfluous	

1. Unwanted and extra hair is called _____ hair.

2. _____ methods of hair removal destroy or damage the hair papilla.

3. The method of permanent hair reduction by electricity is called _____ .

4. With _____ methods of hair removal, repeated treatments are necessary.

5. The method of removing hair by the roots is called _____ .

6. Excessive growth of hair beyond what is normal is called _____ .

7. The presence of excess hair on areas where it is not normally grown is called _____ .

8. The _____ method destroys the hair by decomposing the papilla.

9. The _____ method destroys the hair by coagulating the papilla.

10. A popular group of temporary hair removers are called _____ .

ACTIVITY

Make procedure cards following the procedure sequence taught by your instructor. Use these to practice the proper steps until you are familiar with the sequences of treatments. This activity will instill the proper steps for successful hair removal.

17

ADVANCED ESTHETICS TOPICS:
AN INDUSTRY OVERVIEW

Date: _____

Rating: _____

Text page: 380–399

TOPIC: 1 ADVANCED TREATMENTS

1. Unstable oxygen containing molecules, which are missing an electron, are known as _____
   _____ *Free radicals.* _____.

2. What do free radicals do to the body?

   a) *Damage membranes and normal cellular metabolism systems* _____

   b) *Damage DNA & RNA.* _____

   c) *Contribute to the hardening of Collagen and elastin cells.* _____

   d) _____

3. Vitamin C, Alpha lipoic acid, and DMAE are examples of *Antioxidants* _____.

4. Vitamins, amino acids, and other natural substances can *neutralize* the damaging effects of free radicals.

   a) What can antioxidants do for the skin and body? List five.

      1. _____

      2. _____

      3. _____

      4. _____

      5. _____

5. The process of removing excess accumulations of dead cells from the corneum layers of the epidermis is called:

   a) *Superficial peeling* _____   c) *desquamation* _____

   b) *exfoliation* _____

6. Name several light peels that may be administered by an esthetician.

   a) _____enzyme peels_____

   b) _____Lactic acid_____

   c) _____glycolic acid (30 percent or less)_____

   d) _____Jessner's solution (1 - 3 Coats)_____

7. List the three classifications of light peels.

   a) _____

   b) _____

   c) _____

8. What effects do alphahydroxy acids have on the skin? _____

   _____

9. What factors persuade the CRF (Cell Renewal Factor)?

   a) _____genetics._____

   b) _____natural environment,_____

   c) _____Medical history_____

   d) _____Life style_____

   e) _____personal Care_____

   f) _____natural exfoliation_____

   g) _____physiological desquamation_____

   h) _____accidental desquamation._____

10. Glycolic acids penetrate into the epidermis better because it has the smallest _____molecules_____ size of the AHAs.

11. Peels have many benefits. List eight.

   a) _____improve the texture of the skin_____

   b) _____hydration_____

   c) _____intercellular lipids_____

   d) _____Barrier function_____

   e) _____moisture retention_____

   f) _____elastin_____

   g) _____Collagen production_____

   h) _____Reduce fine lines, Wrinkles, and pigmentation_____

12. List ten conditions that should restrict the use of peels.

   a) _____

   b) _____

   c) _____

   d) _____

   e) _____

   f) _____

   g) _____

   h) _____

   i) _____

   j) _____

13. Clients with acne, sensitive skin, or using Retin-A are good candidates for _enzyme_ peels.

14. Explain the process of menopause and its effect on the skin. _____
_____
_____
_____
_____

15. List eleven ingredients that are helpful for mature skin and rosacea.

a) _Green tea_

b) _Squalane oil_

c) _Sea weed._
Chamomile

d) _micronized Vitamin E_

e) _panthenol - B5._

f) _allantoin_

g) _guarana._

h) _Rose essential oil_

i) _Licorice root._

j) _____

16. An ancient healing practice using essential oils is known as _Aromatherapy._

17. Briefly discuss the benefits of aromatherapy and its relationship to the body's olfactory system.
_____
_____
_____

18. Give the benefits for the following spa services.

a) Body wraps: _____
_____

b) Body polishes: _____

c) Salt glows: _____

d) Body masks: _____

19. Explain the benefits of manual lymph drainage (MLD)._____
_____
_____
_____

20. Long-term age management programs often combine _____ and
_____.

21. Below are definitions of common cosmetic surgical procedures. Place the correct procedure in front of the description.

a) ___Rhinoplastic.___ Surgery that changes the appearance of the nose.

b) ___Rhytidectomy.___ Face lift, removing excess fat, tightens muscles, and removes sagging skin.

c) ___Transconjunctival blepharoplastic___ Surgery to remove bulging fat pads inside the lower eyelid.

d) ___blepharoplastic___ Removes fat and skin from the upper and lower lids.

e) ___Laser resurfacing___ Smoothes wrinkles. Collagen remodeling stimulates growth of new collagen in the dermis.

f) ___abdominoplastic.___ Removes excessive fat deposits and loose skin from the abdomen to tuck and tighten the area.

g) ___Mammoplastic___ Breast surgery to enlarge or reduce, or to reconstruct breasts.

h) ___Liposuction.___ Surgically removes fat pockets.

WORD REVIEW

ayurvedic	endermology	olfactory system
balneotherapy	hydrotherapy	phenol
botox	lancets	TCA
collagen	nonablative	

RAPID REVIEW TEST

Date: _____

Rating: _____

Insert the correct term in the space provided.

acne	free radicals	phytotherapy
aplha lipoic acid	hydrotherapy	rosacea
botox	light peels	salicylic acid
endermology	manual lymph drainage	salt glows
fibroblasts	olfactory system	

1. An antioxidant that is water and oil soluble and found in every cell in the body is _____ ___alpha lipoic acid___ .

2. A disorder resulting in couperose veins and congestion of the skin is known as ___Rosacea___ .

3. Glycolic acid, lactic acid, salicylic acid, and azelaic acid are types of peels appropriate for _____acne_____ skin.

4. Cells found in collagen and elastin are called _____fibroblasts_____.

5. Skin care formulas are designed to combat _____free radicals_____.

6. An esthetician uses procedures designed to penetrate only the epidermis and are known as _____light peels_____.

7. _____Salicylic acid_____ is derived from willow bark and wintergreen.

8. _____manual lymph drainage_____ is a procedure that stimulates lymph fluid to flow through the lymphatic vessels.

9. Aromatherapy uses oils and herbs to affect the body's _____olfactory system_____.

10. The treatment of cellulite is called _____Endermology_____.

11. A spa treatment that uses ice and steam is referred to as _____hydrotherapy_____.

12. A serum made from the bacteria *Clostridium botulinum* is called _____Botox_____.

13. The use of plant extracts for therapeutic benefits is called _____phytotherapy_____.

14. Exfoliation treatments using sea salt and oil or lotions are called _____salt glows_____.

18

THE WORLD OF MAKEUP

Date _____

Rating _____

Text pages: 400–454

TOPIC 1: INTRODUCTION TO MAKEUP AND ITS PURPOSE

1. Knowledge of color theory, analyzing facial features, and corrective makeup techniques are all part of being a successful makeup artist.

   a) What is the main purpose of makeup? _____

   _____

   b) Name two other benefits of makeup on our "inner-self"?

   1. _____

   2. _____

   c) In addition to working in spas, list four other avenues a makeup artist might consider.

   1. _____   3. _____

   2. _____   4. _____

2. Makeup comes in many forms for the needs of the total look.

   a) For each type listed below, give an example in the space provided.

   1. Bottles—_____   4. Sticks—_____

   2. Tubes—_____   5. Wands—_____

   3. Powders—_____   6. Creams—_____

3. What is the purpose of foundation? List three benefits of its use.

   a) _____

   b) _____

   c) _____

4. Complete the following sentences with the list of words provided.

cream   oil-free

liquid   powder

a) _____Powder_____ foundations consist of a base mixed with pigment, and are good for oily skin.

b) _____Cream_____ foundations are generally suited for oily to normal skin and give medium to heavier coverage.

c) _____Liquid_____ foundations are used on oily to normal skin, giving sheer to medium coverage.

d) _____Oil-free_____ foundations are water-based and are free of mineral oil.

5. What determines the color selection of foundations? _____Skintone_____

a) The three colors of warm-toned skin are _____yellow, orange or red orange_____.

b) Cool-toned skin generally appears as _____.

6. When selecting foundation colors, where is the foundation tested to be sure it will blend well with the client's natural skin color? _____Jawline._____

7. Why are concealers used in makeup applications? _____

_____

a) Why is it important to match concealer color to skin color? _____

_____

8. Powders will add a _____matte_____ or _____dull_____ finish to the face, and will also conceal minor discolorations.

a) The two types of powders are _____loose_____ and _____pressed_____.

b) The general purpose of using face powder is to _____set the makeup._____.

9. _____Blush_____ and _____rouge_____ are other terms used for cheek color.

a) List two reasons cheek color is used during a makeup application.

1. _____it gives a natural-looking glow_____

2. _____Helps to create more attractive facial contours_____

b) What are the specific ingredients used to make an oil-based cheek color water resistant?

1. _____   3. _____

2. _____   4. _____

c) Cheek color comes in a variety of consistencies. List two formulas and include the skin type (dry, normal, oily) for which it is best suited.

1. _____   _____

2. _____   _____

10. Eye shadows _____ and _____ the eyes and are available in endless colors.

a) What is a common mistake when choosing a color of eye shadow? _____
_____

b) A _____ shade will make the natural color of the iris appear lighter.

c) Eye makeup color may match the client's _____ .

d) What are the three categories of eye shadow colors and what is their purpose during a makeup application?

1. _____   _____

2. _____   _____

3. _____   _____

11. The common forms of eyeliner are _____ , _____ ,
_____ , and _____ .

a) Eyeliner applied to the inner rim of the eyes can cause infection to the tear duct, and lead to *causing tearing* , *burning of vision* , and *permanent pigmentation of the mucous membrane lining the inside of the eye .*

b) What is the proper procedure for applying powdered eyeliner? _____
_____

c) To ensure a smooth application of eyeliner, what course of action may you use? _____
_____

12. Why is eyebrow color used during a makeup application? _____
It is suggested to _____ harsh contrasts between the color of hair and eyebrow color.

13. List the ingredients of mascara.

a) *water*   d) *film-formers*

b) *wax*   e) *preservatives .*

c) *thickeners*

14. a) What are the inert pigments used to give mascara its color?

1. _Carbon Black_   4. _chromium oxide_

2. _Carmine_   5. _iron oxides._

3. _ultramarine_

b) What is the common injury you want to avoid when applying mascara? _poking the eye with the applicator_

15. Lip color comes in various forms. List five.

a) _cream_   d) _gels._

b) _glosses_   e) _sticks._

c) _pencils_

16. When choosing a lip color, what should you take into consideration? List four.

a) _eye color_   c) _lip shape_

b) _skin tone_   d) _____

17. Lip liners are used to keep lip color from _feathering_ .

18. _____ is used for theatrical makeup applications.

19. When covering scars or applying makeup for video shoots, a _____ makeup works best.

20. Give the purpose of the makeup brushes listed below.

Powder brush _for Blending._

Concealer brush _Blemishes._

Blush brush _powder Blush._

Lip brush _Apply Concealer._

Eye shadow brush _____

Lash and brow brush _remove excess mascara or to comb brows_

WORD REVIEW

Annetto	emulsion	iridescent
corrective	enhance	minimize
coverage	fluorescent	petroleum
diminish	illusion	pigmentation
dramatic	incandescent	
emphasize	inert	

RAPID REVIEW TEST

Date:_____

Rating: _____

Insert the correct term in the space provided.

alcohol	demarcation	subtle
before	disposable	surfactants
camouflage	face shape	sanitized
concealers	lip colors	thickening
darkening	mascara	wipe
defining	reshape	

1. Natural skin tone, hair and eye color, and _____ should be considered when choosing makeup.

2. _____ makeup is used in minimizing disfigurements.

3. A line of _____ should never be visible when applying foundations.

4. _____ should be used sparingly, and blended on the edges for a natural look.

5. Mascara finishes the eyelashes by _____ , _____ , and _____ them.

6. _____ enable cream cheek colors to penetrate the hair follicles and cracks of the skin.

7. The choice of eye shadow colors should be more _____ for daytime wear.

8. The pencil sharpener should be _____ after each use to avoid contamination.

9. It is important to _____ the sharpened pencil with a tissue, to remove loose particles.

10. _____ is considered as a polymer product.

11. If using an eyelash curler, this procedure must be completed _____ applying mascara.

12. _____ are a great source of retail.

13. _____ will break down natural bristles and dry brushes over time.

14. When drying brushes, it is important to _____ the bristles to the proper contour.

15. A _____ wand is used when applying mascara to avoid double-dipping.

TOPIC 2: MAKEUP COLOR THEORY

1. _____ , _____ , and _____ are considered primary colors. What separates these colors from all other colors? _____

2. How are secondary colors created? _____
   _____ , _____ , and _____ are the three secondary colors.

3. Tertiary colors are obtained by mixing equal amounts of a secondary color with its _____ neighbor. By using a color wheel, create six tertiary colors.

   a) _____   d) _____

   b) _____   e) _____

   c) _____   f) _____

4. How are neutral colors created from primary and secondary colors? _____
   _____

5. a) How do you create a greater contrast between colors? _____
   _____

   b) Create three scenarios of contrast using a color wheel.

      1. _____

      2. _____

      3. _____

6. a) Colors are classified as _____ , neutral, or cool. What is distinctive of warm tones?
   _____

b) Cool tones have what characteristic? _____

c) What two colors can be considered warm and cool? _____

_____

7. What three factors must you take into consideration when choosing makeup colors?

a) _____

b) _____

c) _____

8. Answer the following questions by writing "true" or "false" in the space provided.

a) _____   Medium skin is always considered neutral.

b) _____   Dark skin will require a warm tone to create a balanced look.

c) _____   Skin color is created by blood showing through the skin.

d) _____   To create dramatic eyes, you should use the same color of eye shadow as the eye color.

e) _____   Light skin can be warm, cool, or neutral.

f) _____   Blue colors are complementary to most skin colors.

g) _____   Purple eye shadow will blend well with blemished skin.

h) _____   Red will disguise freckles.

i) _____   To avoid a chalky or gray look, it is best to use lighter colors.

9. List seven common choices of color to complement blue eyes.

a) _____   e) _____

b) _____   f) _____

c) _____   g) _____

d) _____

10. To complement green eyes, list six colors that are commonly used.

a) _____   d) _____

b) _____   e) _____

c) _____   f) _____

11. Brown eyes are considered as _____ and can support any color.

12. Certain colors can have adverse appearances. Describe the appearance with using red or orange on the eyes. _____

13. If warm and cool colors are combined with eye shadow, cheek and lip color, what is the result?

_____

14. After choosing complementing colors for eyes and skin tone, why should you consider hair color?

_____

_____

TOPIC 3: FACE SHAPES AND PROPORTIONS

1. The general rule when applying makeup is to _____ the attractive features and _____ the less attractive ones.

2. List the seven facial shapes.

   a) _____   e) _____

   b) _____   f) _____

   c) _____   g) _____

   d) _____

3. Write the corrective makeup application for the following features.

   a) Protruding forehead _____

   b) Low forehead _____

   c) Large nose _____

   d) Round eyes _____

   e) Heavy-lidded _____

   f) Deep-set eyes _____

   g) Dark circles under the eyes _____

4. On the following diagrams, use colored pencils or crayons to shade the eyes and lips to best enhance or correct the irregularities.

Eye Shapes

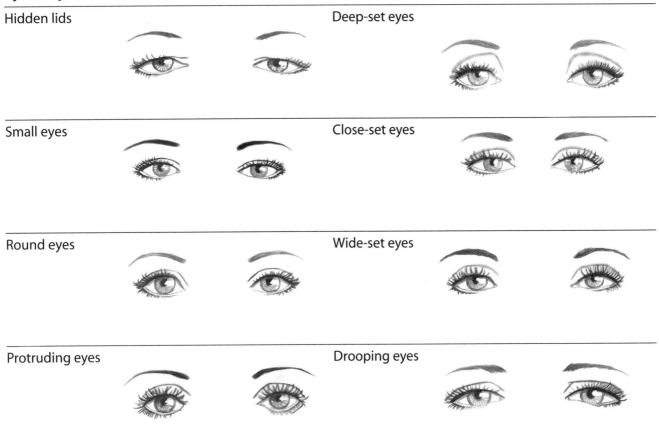

Hidden lids	Deep-set eyes
Small eyes	Close-set eyes
Round eyes	Wide-set eyes
Protruding eyes	Drooping eyes

Lip Shape	Line	Color
Thin lower lip		
Thin upper lip		
Thin upper and lower lips		

(continued)

Lip Shape		**Line**	**Color**
Cupid bow or pointed upper lip			
Large full lips			
Small mouth and lips			
Drooping corners			
Uneven lips			
Straight upper lip			
Fine lines around the lips			

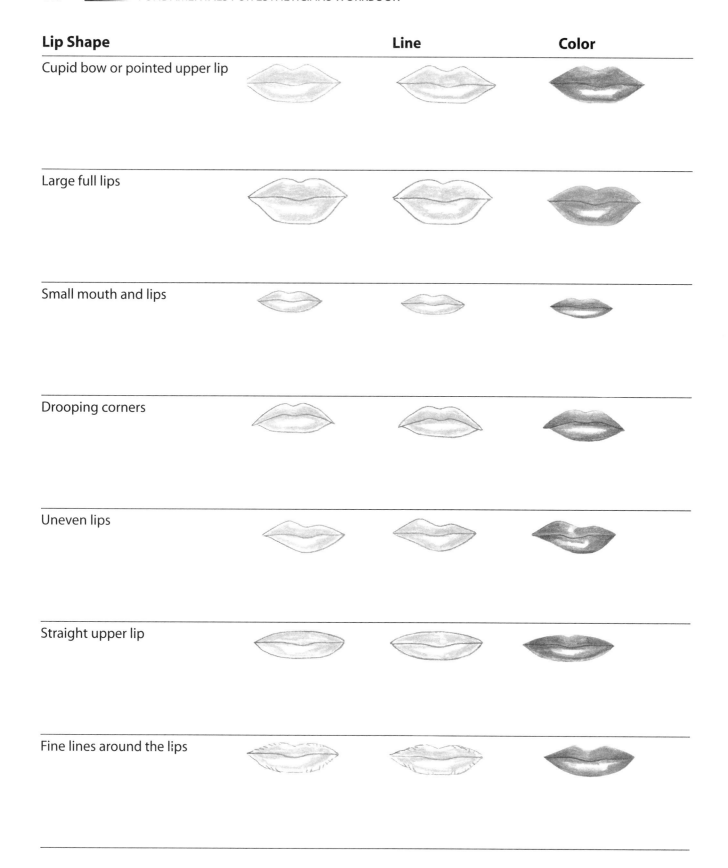

5. Describe the method of determining eyebrow shape. _____

    _____

    _____

    _____

    _____

    _____

6. To correct a ruddy complexion, what color of foundation should be used? _____

7. A skin tone that has a yellowish hue requires a _____ -based foundation to neutralize the tone.

8. During the consultation, there is specific information that should be gathered. List seven items to be discussed with your client.

    a) _____

    b) _____

    c) _____

    d) _____

    e) _____

    f) _____

    g) _____

9. Why is it important to use correct lighting? _____

    _____

    _____

WORD REVIEW

complementary	illusion	ruddy
contour	incandescent	sallow
cool	inverted	secondary
emphasize	minimize	subdue
enhance	neutral	translucent
fluorescent	pigment	tertiary
harmony	primary	vertical
horizontal	proportional	warm

RAPID REVIEW TEST

Date: _____

Rating: _____

Insert the correct term in the space provided. Some terms may be used more than once.

complementary	inverted triangle	round
diamond	light	shadowing
flat	neutral	square
highlighting	pear	three-fourths
horizontal	pigmentation	warm
intensity		

1. Colors located directly opposite each other on the color wheel are called _____ colors.

2. Colors are categorized as warm, cool, and _____.

3. _____ is the degree of purity or brilliance of colors.

4. Skin color is determined by the amount of _____ in the skin.

5. Dark colors used on _____ skin will create a dramatic look.

6. To emphasize color effectively, it is suggested to use _____ colors.

7. _____ and cool colors mixed on a face creates an unbalanced appearance.

8. The face is divided into three _____ sections for the purpose of determining proportions.

9. A _____ face is broader in proportion to its length.

10. A square jawline and wide forehead are characteristic of a _____ face.

11. The ideal face is approximately _____ wide as it is long.

12. A facial shape with the jawline wider than the forehead is classified as an _____ or _____ shape.

13. A _____ -shaped face is its widest at the cheekbones.

14. In makeup, _____ emphasizes, while _____ minimizes.

15. It is best to use _____ lip color on large, full lips.

TOPIC 4: SUPPLIES AND APPLICATION OF MAKEUP

1. To apply foundation and concealer, a _____ is most effective because of its versatility.

2. What should be used to apply mascara? _____

3. _____ can be used for quick fixes or correcting mistakes.

4. What are the four general steps in a complete makeup application?

   a) _____   c) _____

   b) _____   d) _____

5. Why is lifting the eye skin not recommended? _____
_____
_____

6. Products must be _____ to give the makeup service a professional, finished look.

7. During an application for a special event that will be in subdued light, it is important to remember to use more _____ in the application.

8. What are two special effects that you might use for a special occasion?

   a) _____   b) _____

9. If every feature is intensified, the end result will appear _____.

10. Why is it necessary to apply more product for photography and film/video applications? _____
_____

11. What applications require the most exaggerated type of application? _____
_____

12. What are the two types of artificial eyelashes? _____

   a) Give the other name for applying individual eyelashes. _____

ACTIVITY

Create a dialog that can be used during your consultation that includes all of the information that you need. Write it in a way that it will interact with your client, using open-ended questions, not just yes or no questions. Try it on a classmate and document the conversation to see if you did indeed receive all of the information necessary for a complete consultation.

Create a closure dialog that includes a retail segment. Retail can be an important part of your income. Practicing while in school will ensure that you have a solid understanding of how to sell. There is not an exact dialog for use on all clients, so begin simple, with one item, and increase each time. There is a great deal of psychology in selling techniques, and there are many articles for your self-study.

19

THE SALON/SPA BUSINESS

Date: _____

Rating: _____

Text pages: 457–493

TOPIC 1: SUCCEEDING IN A SERVICE PROFESSION

1. Professional skin care today integrates the principles not only of beauty but also of health and _____
   _____ .

2. The fastest-growing segment of the U.S. population is the so-called _____ .

3. What are three factors that have fueled the current client demand for anti-aging treatments and _____
   products?

   a) _____

   b) _____

   c) _____

4. List seven qualities and behaviors that help you provide client-focused services.

   a) _____

   b) _____

   c) _____

   d) _____

   e) _____

   f) _____

   g) _____

5. When you work for a salon, you must learn to put its needs and those of its _____
   ahead of your personal concerns.

6. Businesses provide written statements of their policies and procedures in the form of _____
   _____ or _____ .

7. What are two reasons that some salons dictate exactly how certain procedures should be performed?

   a) _____

   _____

   b) _____

   _____

8. Name six ways you can ensure your clients' safety and protect yourself and the salon from liability problems.

   a) _____

   b) _____

   c) _____

   d) _____

   e) _____

   _____

   f) _____

   _____

9. Because you may be held liable in case of accidents, it may be a good idea to obtain an additional

   _____.

10. To be a good team player, each employee must be:

   a) _____

   b) _____

   c) _____

   d) _____

   e) _____

   f) _____

11. Describe the positive aspects of being evaluated by your employer. _____

   _____

   _____

12. Asking your employer for suggestions on how to do your job better demonstrates that you are mature enough to handle _____ criticism.

TOPIC 2: GOING INTO BUSINESS FOR YOURSELF

1. Define *booth rental*. _____

   _____

   _____

   _____

2. List five advantages of renting a booth in a salon.

   a) _____

   b) _____

   c) _____

   d) _____

   e) _____

3. List five disadvantages of booth rental.

   a) _____

   b) _____

   c) _____

   d) _____

   e) _____

4. What factors must enter into a decision about where to locate a salon or spa?

   a) _____

   b) _____

   c) _____

5. What are demographics? How can a knowledge of the demographics of an area be helpful in deciding where to locate a business? _____

   _____

   _____

   _____

   _____

6. It is possible for similar businesses to exist next to each other successfully if they target _____

   _____ .

7. Because of potential competition, it is important before opening a business in any area to thoroughly

   _____ .

8. A _____ provides you with a map or blueprint that can guide you in making informed decisions.

9. List some of the information that should be included in a business plan.

   a) _____

   b) _____

   c) _____

   _____

10. Define these terms:

    a) fixed costs   _____

    b) variable costs _____

    c) revenue   _____

    d) profit   _____

11. List fourteen factors that should be kept in mind as a salon layout is planned.

    a) _____

    b) _____

    c) _____

    d) _____

    e) _____

    f) _____

    g) _____

    h) _____

    i) _____

    j) _____

    k) _____

    l) _____

m) _____

n) _____

12. In some states there are levels of _____ that may require a practitioner to work under another, more experienced professional for a certain period of time before operating independently.

13. Sales tax, licenses, and employee compensation are regulated by the _____ .

14. Building renovations and business codes are supervised by _____ .

15. The federal government oversees laws regarding:

    a) _____

    b) _____

    c) _____

16. One insurance obligation required by law is _____ compensation.

17. The government agency that oversees workplace safety is _____

    _____ .

18. Name and describe briefly the three different kinds of business ownership.

    a) _____

    _____

    _____

    _____

    b) _____

    _____

    _____

    _____

    c) _____

    _____

    _____

    _____

19. Before buying an established salon—and for many other transactions—it is a good idea to consult professionals such as _____ and _____ .

20. List five ways you can protect your business against fire, theft, and lawsuits.

    a) _____

    b) _____

    c) _____

    d) _____

    e) _____

    _____

21. One aspect of good money management is determining how much capital you will need to operate your salon for at least _____ years.

22. When you price the services your salon offers, you should know what your clients want and value as well as _____ .

23. To develop smooth and harmonious working relationships in the salon, a manager must:

    a) _____

    b) _____

    c) _____

24. Salon policies concerning such problems as cancellations, no-shows, and product returns should be posted in an area that is extremely _____ .

25. Why is it important to keep accurate records pertaining to your business?

    a) _____

    b) _____

    c) _____

26. Canceled checks and payroll, monthly, and yearly records should generally be held for at least _____ _____ years.

27. Keeping a careful track of inventory helps you:

    a) _____

    b) _____

    c) _____

    d) _____

28. Name and define the two categories of inventory.

a) _____

b) _____

TOPIC 3: OPERATING A SUCCESSFUL SKIN CARE BUSINESS

1. Clients form their first impression of a salon in the _____ .

2. What are the primary functions of the receptionist?

a) _____

b) _____

c) _____

d) _____

e) _____

f) _____

3. What kind of information must a receptionist be prepared to give clients? _____

_____

_____

4. The receptionist can help everyone stay on schedule by being careful not to _____ .

5. The lifeline of salon operations is still considered to be the _____ .

6. List nine guidelines for telephone etiquette in the salon.

a) _____

b) _____

c) _____

d) _____

e) _____

f) _____

g) _____

h) _____

i) _____

_____

7. Name the factors you should consider when evaluating prospective employees.

a) _____   d) _____

b) _____   e) _____

c) _____   f) _____

8. What is a job description? _____
_____

9. Job descriptions help employees understand what is expected of them, and also provide a standard for
_____ .

10. What is the difference between an employee manual and a procedural guide? _____
_____
_____
_____
_____
_____

11. List nine guidelines for establishing good employee relations.

a) _____

b) _____

c) _____

d) _____

e) _____

f) _____

g) _____

h) _____

i) _____

12. Define *public relations*. _____
_____

ACTIVITY

Design a salon that will serve men and women, keeping in mind that privacy is needed. Describe the color scheme, décor, etc. Design the gowns that will be used for protecting clothing. What music, if any, will be playing? How do you feel that this plan will promote a unisex salon?

20

SELLING PRODUCTS AND SERVICES

Date _____

Rating_____

Text pages: 494–521

TOPIC 1: SELLING IN THE SALON

1. Why is selling in the salon the esthetician's professional responsibility? _____
   _____
   _____

2. Explain the concept of consultative selling. _____
   _____
   _____
   _____

3. List eight principles of selling.

   a) _____

   b) _____

   c) _____

   d) _____

   e) _____

   f) _____

   g) _____

   h) _____
   _____

4. If a client is unsure about a treatment or product, the esthetician should _____
   _____
   _____

5. In the salon, selling is the responsibility of _____.

6. Define *upselling services.* _____
   _____

7. Define *retailing* as it is practiced in the salon. _____

_____

8. How can estheticians confidently make product recommendations for their clients? _____

_____

_____

_____

9. What five steps can you take to better understand and recommend various products?

a) _____

b) _____

_____

c) _____

d) _____

e) _____

TOPIC 2: UNDERSTANDING CLIENT NEEDS AND RETAINING CLIENTS

1. The questionnaire or _____ is an important tool that allows the esthetician to learn about a client's overall skin condition.

2. Client questionnaires should include medical information such as known _____ or sensitivities as well as the use of any drugs or _____ .

3. Explain the function of client records. _____

_____

_____

4. In addition to the client's name, address, and telephone number, what kinds of information can be included in client records?

a) _____   e) _____

b) _____   f) _____

c) _____   g) _____

d) _____

5. In a service industry such as esthetics, the most important strategy for high client retention is _____

_____ .

6. List five guidelines that can help an esthetician ensure client satisfaction and retention.

   a) _____

   b) _____

   c) _____

   d) _____

   e) _____

7. The first step in educating a client is understanding _____ .

8. A common mistake is to give the client too much information during the _____ process, rather than during the skin analysis or closing consultation.

9. If a client asks you about a product or procedure that is not available at your salon, you should _____ _____ .

TOPIC 3: MARKETING

1. What is marketing? _____
   _____

2. Advertising and direct marketing are methods of _____ .

3. List ten ways to promote products and services in the salon.

   a) _____

   b) _____

   c) _____

   d) _____

   e) _____

   f) _____

   g) _____

   h) _____

   i) _____

   j) _____

4. Broadly speaking, any activity that promotes the salon or spa can be called _____ .

5. The best form of advertising is a _____ .

6. Define *advertising*. _____

_____

7. On average, a new business might spend _____ of total projected revenues on advertising, while an established business might spend _____ .

8. Match the following forms of advertising with their descriptions.

    classified advertising   magazines   radio and television

    direct mail   newspapers

a) _____ more expensive methods, reach large numbers of consumers, require consistent efforts to be effective

b) _____ generally less expensive, usually uses text only

c) _____ good way to target potential clients and reach existing customers, uses mailing lists and databases

d) _____ somewhat pricier than newspapers, good way to reach specific target market

e) _____ cost-effective method that reaches a large number of consumers; may use graphics

9. Press releases, participation in special events, and volunteering the salon's services for good causes are ways to gain _____ or free media attention.

TOPIC 4: BUILDING A CLIENTELE

1. A new client must leave the salon with two reasons for wanting to return:

a) _____

_____

b) _____

2. It is _____ clients that keep a salon business going.

3. When you are friendly and courteous with clients but do not socialize with them or give personal advice, you are maintaining appropriate professional _____ .

4. List six ways the salon can expand its network of referrals.

a) _____

b) _____

c) _____

d) _____

e) _____

f) _____

TOPIC 5: PRESENTING YOUR PRODUCTS AND SERVICES

1. One of the more expensive printed materials a salon invests in is the brochure or _____
_____ .

2. A brochure should reflect both the salon's image and its _____ .

3. Retail product displays should be both _____ and attractive.

4. Retail displays should blend with the _____ of the salon rather than compete
for attention.

TOPIC 6: CLOSING THE SALE

1. The closing _____ is a good time for the esthetician and the client to review the
client's concerns and discuss a home-care program.

2. The best way to help clients remember instructions for at-home skin care is to _____
_____ .

3. If a client does not wish to buy all the products the esthetician recommends, the esthetician should not
be forceful but rather focus on building the client's _____ first.

4. The most effective way to follow up a treatment with a client is with a _____ .

5. Clients who receive more aggressive treatments should be called within _____ , while
those who are starting a new home-care regimen should be called within _____ . All
other clients should be called within _____ .

21

CAREER PLANNING

Date: _____

Rating: _____

Text pages: 522–560

TOPIC 1: GOALS AND LONG-TERM PLANNING

1. One of the first steps in developing long-term goals is to define your _____

_____ .

2. Name and briefly define the three key elements that contribute to your professional image.

   a) _____

   _____

   b) _____

   _____

   c) _____

   _____

3. List nine ways in which you can demonstrate a good work ethic.

   a) _____

   b) _____

   c) _____

   d) _____

   e) _____

   f) _____

   g) _____

   h) _____

   i) _____

4. The first step in effective time management is _____ .

5. What kinds of tasks can you perform at the end of the day in preparation for the next day's workload?

a) _____

b) _____

c) _____

d) _____

e) _____

f) _____

6. Careful planning and preparation help ensure that the service is _____ , which is one of the perceived benefits for clients.

TOPIC 2: PREPARING FOR LICENSURE

1. Before you can apply for your first job, you must complete the required training and _____
_____ .

2. List nine strategies for preparing for your licensing exam.

a) _____

b) _____

c) _____

d) _____

e) _____

f) _____

g) _____

h) _____

i) _____
_____

3. Match the following types of test questions with their descriptions.

essay   multiple choice
matching   true or false

_____ offer only two choices

_____ match questions to a list of choices

_____ typically offer four to six choices

_____ open-ended questions that allow testers flexibility in how they present their answer

4. True or false questions using absolute words such as *all*, *none*, *always*, or *never* are generally _____ _____ .

5. In multiple-choice questions, two choices that are identical must both be _____ .

6. Before you begin a test, if something is not clear, always _____ .

7. In a written exam, answer questions you are _____ about first, and save the questions you are _____ about for last.

8. When taking a trial run for a practical exam, pay close attention to timing as well as to _____ _____ .

9. Your _____ gives potential employers a summary of your education, work experience, and relevant accomplishments and achievements.

10. When you compose your resume, remember that the average employer will spend about _____ seconds scanning it to decide whether or not to contact you for an interview.

11. What general types of information should you include in your resume?

a) _____

b) _____

c) _____

d) _____

e) _____

12. Your resume should highlight _____ skills, that is, skills that can be applied from other work experiences.

13. Words such as *established, increased,* and *developed* are considered _____ words.

14. List four things you should *not* include in a resume.

a) _____

b) _____

c) _____

d) _____

15. A resume should always be accompanied by a _____ that completes the written presentation of your work.

16. An effective cover letter includes:

a) _____

b) _____

c) _____

d) _____

17. A _____ of your work includes before and after photos of your skin care or makeup artistry, awards, letters of recognition, and other documents.

TOPIC 3: THE JOB SEARCH

1. Before accepting a job offer it is a good idea to learn as much as you can about a salon's _____ and _____.

2. List six work conditions that you should consider when searching for the right job fit.

a) _____

b) _____

c) _____

d) _____

e) _____

f) _____

3. If you wish to stay abreast of new treatments and techniques, you may wish to find out if a prospective employer offers _____ .

4. A good way to learn about a salon or spa without the pressure of being a job candidate is an _____
_____ .

5. Professional etiquette dictates that you send a handwritten _____
to a salon owner or manager who meets with you.

6. Identify the types of skin care practice described below.

_____ provides hair, nail, and skin care services

_____ focuses on health; may offer skin care and holistic services targeted to healthy aging

_____ integrates surgical and esthetic skin care treatments and spa services

_____ offers variety of skin care treatments for face and body, makeup, nail care, massage, and other holistic services

7. In what types of settings are medi-spas located?

a) _____

b) _____

c) _____

8. A _____ salon is owned by individuals who pay a fee to use the company name and is part of a larger organization or chain of salons.

9. Who makes decisions about size, location, and services in a franchise? _____

10. What are two advantages to belonging to a franchise? _____
_____

11. What are three advantages of working for an independently owned skin care clinic or day spa?

a) _____

b) _____

c) _____

12. What are three advantages of working for a full-service salon or day spa?

a) _____

b) _____

c) _____

_____

13. The _____ or _____ spa is often associated with a hotel facility.

14. Define *networking*. _____

_____

15. Always take an additional copy of your _____ to a job interview even if you have already mailed one to the interviewer.

16. Describe briefly how each of the following elements should fit into your overall appearance on a job interview:

a) makeup _____

b) nails _____

c) hairstyle _____

d) clothing _____

17. List nine basic guidelines for an effective job interview.

a) _____

b) _____

c) _____

d) _____

e) _____

f) _____

g) _____

h) _____

i) _____

18. What are some questions that you cannot legally be asked during an interview? _____

_____

_____

TOPIC 4: ON THE JOB

1. Estheticians may be required to educate not only clients but also _____ about new treatments and products.

2. A good standard for evaluating an employee's performance is the _____.

3. Explain the quota system. _____

_____

4. Many salon managers set both individual and _____ sales goals.

5. An esthetician is generally evaluated _____ after beginning a job and once a year thereafter.

6. The salon industry bases its wage structure largely on a percentage or _____ method.

7. What are the factors that affect wages?

    a) _____

    b) _____

    c) _____

    d) _____

8. Salaries based on a _____ rate are generally based on a minimum wage and a 40-hour week, even if you work more hours.

9. Salaries based on an _____ rate are paid only for the hours you work.

10. _____ -based wages are tied directly to your performance and vary between _____ and _____ percent of the services you perform.

11. The first step in financial planning is keeping track of all your _____ and weighing them against your total _____.

12. Meeting your financial obligations in a timely fashion helps you establish good _____, which is a particularly important consideration if you wish to own your own business someday.

TOPIC 5: COMMUNICATION SKILLS

1. Esthetics is a _____ -oriented business that requires learning to _____ effectively with others.

2. List ten guidelines for effective communication.

   a) _____

   b) _____

   c) _____

   d) _____

   e) _____

   f) _____

   g) _____

   h) _____

   i) _____

   j) _____

3. What is a role model? _____

   _____

4. List seven sources of continuing and advanced education.

   a) _____

   b) _____

   c) _____

   d) _____

   e) _____

   f) _____

   g) _____